T0259445

Ankle Arthritis

Guest Editor

JESSE B. BURKS, DPM, MS, FACFAS

CLINICS IN PODIATRIC MEDICINE AND SURGERY

www.podiatric.theclinics.com

Consulting Editor
THOMAS ZGONIS, DPM, FACFAS

October 2012 • Volume 29 • Number 4

SAUNDERS an imprint of ELSEVIER, Inc.

W.B. SAUNDERS COMPANY
A Division of Elsevier Inc.

1600 John F. Kennedy Boulevard • Suite 1800 • Philadelphia, Pennsylvania 19103-2899

http://www.theclinics.com

CLINICS IN PODIATRIC MEDICINE AND SURGERY Volume 29, Number 4
October 2012 ISSN 0891-8422, ISBN-13: 978-1-4557-4944-7

Editor: Patrick Manley

Clinics in Podiatric Medicine and Surgery (ISSN 0891-8422) is published quarterly by Elsevier Inc., 360 Park Avenue South, New York, NY 10010-1710. Months of issue are January, April, July, and October. Business and Editorial Offices: 1600 John F. Kennedy Blvd., Ste. 1800, Philadelphia, PA 19103-2899. Customer Service Office: 3251 Riverport Lane, Maryland Heights, MO 63043. Periodicals postage paid at NewYork, NY and additional mailing offices. Subscription prices are $292.00 per year for US individuals, $410.00 per year for US institutions, $148.00 per year for US students and residents, $350.00 per year for Canadian individuals, $508.00 for Canadian institutions, $415.00 for international individuals, $508.00 per year for international institutions and $208.00 per year for Canadian and foreign students/residents. To receive student/resident rate, orders must be accompanied by name of affiliated institution, date of term, and the *signature* of program/residency coordinator on institution letterhead. Orders will be billed at individual rate until proof of status is received. Foreign air speed delivery is included in all *Clinics* subscription prices. All prices are subject to change without notice. POSTMASTER: Send address changes to *Clinics in Podiatric Medicine and Surgery*, Elsevier Health Sciences Division, Subscription Customer Service, 3251 Riverport Lane, Maryland Heights, MO 63043. **Customer Service: 1-800-654-2452 (US). From outside of the US, call 314-447-8871. Fax: 314-447-8029. E-mail: JournalsCustomerService-usa@elsevier.com (for print support); JournalsOnlineSupport-usa@elsevier.com (for online support).**

Reprints. For copies of 100 or more of articles in this publication, please contact the Commercial Reprints Department, Elsevier Inc., 360 Park Avenue South, New York, NY 10010-1710. Tel.: 212-633-3812; Fax: 212-462-1935; E-mail: reprints@elsevier.com.

Clinics in Podiatric Medicine and Surgery is covered in *MEDLINE/PubMed (Index Medicus) and EMBASE/Excerpta Medica.*

Printed and bound by CPI Group (UK) Ltd, Croydon, CR0 4YY

Transferred to digital print 2012

CLINICS IN PODIATRIC MEDICINE AND SURGERY

CONSULTING EDITOR
THOMAS ZGONIS, DPM, FACFAS

Contributors

CONSULTING EDITOR

THOMAS ZGONIS, DPM, FACFAS
Director, Podiatric Surgical Residency and Reconstructive Fellowship Programs;
Chief, Division of Podiatric Medicine and Surgery; Associate Professor, Department
of Orthopedic Surgery, The University of Texas Health Science Center at San Antonio,
San Antonio, Texas

GUEST EDITOR

JESSE B. BURKS, DPM, MS, FACFAS
OrthoSurgeons, Little Rock, Arkansas

AUTHORS

BRANDON BORER, DPM
Indianapolis, Indiana

JESSE B. BURKS, DPM, MS, FACFAS
OrthoSurgeons, Little Rock, Arkansas

SHIRLEY M. CATOIRE, DPM, AACFAS
Indianapolis, Indiana

DAVINA CROSS, DPM
Resident, Heritage Valley Health Systems, Beaver, Pennsylvania

PATRICK A. DEHEER, DPM, FACFAS
Franklin, Indiana

LAWRENCE A. DIDOMENICO, DPM, FACFAS
Section Chief, Departments of Podiatry and Surgery, St. Elizabeth Health Center; Private
Practice, The Ankle and Foot Care Centers, Youngstown, Ohio

ZACHARIA FACAROS, DPM
Weil Foot & Ankle Institute, Des Plaines, Illinois

JOHN E. HERZENBERG, MD
Director, International Center for Limb Lengthening/Rubin Institute for Advanced
Orthopedics, Sinai Hospital of Baltimore, Baltimore, Maryland

BRADLEY M. LAMM, DPM, FACFAS
Head of the Foot and Ankle Surgery Director, Foot and Ankle Deformity Correction
Fellowship, International Center for Limb Lengthening/Rubin Institute for Advanced
Orthopedics, Sinai Hospital of Baltimore, Baltimore, Maryland

BRADLEY A. LEVITT, DPM
Clinical Instructor and Fellow in Reconstructive Foot and Ankle Surgery, Division of Podiatric Medicine and Surgery, Department of Orthopaedic Surgery, University of Texas Health Science Center at San Antonio, San Antonio, Texas

BENJAMIN D. OVERLEY Jr, DPM, FACFAS
Foot and Ankle Specialist, PMSI Orthopedics, Pottstown, Pennsylvania

CRYSTAL L. RAMANUJAM, DPM, MSc
Assistant Professor, Division of Podiatric Medicine and Surgery, Department of Orthopaedic Surgery, University of Texas Health Science Center at San Antonio, San Antonio, Texas

BRYAN A. SAGRAY, DPM
Clinical Instructor and Fellow in Reconstructive Foot and Ankle Surgery, Division of Podiatric Medicine and Surgery, Department of Orthopaedic Surgery, University of Texas Health Science Center at San Antonio, San Antonio, Texas

JASON L. SEITER, DPM, FACFAS
Fort Smith, Arkansas

KENNETH P. SEITER Jr, DPM, AACFAS
Fort Smith, Arkansas

NOMAN A. SIDDIQUI, DPM, MHA, AACFAS
Fellow, Foot and Ankle Deformity Correction, International Center for Limb Lengthening/ Rubin Institute for Advanced Orthopedics, Sinai Hospital of Baltimore, Baltimore, Maryland

JESSICA TAULMAN, DPM
Indianapolis, Indiana

THOMAS ZGONIS, DPM, FACFAS
Associate Professor, Fellowship Director in Reconstructive Foot and Ankle Surgery and Chief, Division of Podiatric Medicine and Surgery, Department of Orthopaedic Surgery, University of Texas Health Science Center at San Antonio, San Antonio, Texas

Contents

> Ankle replacement systems have not been as reliable as hip replacements
> in providing long-term relief of pain, increased motion, and return to full
> activity. Supramalleolar Osteotomy is an extraarticular procedure that re-
> aligns the mechanical axis, thereby restoring ankle function. The literature
> discussing knee arthritis has shown that realignment osteotomies of the
> tibia improve function and prolong total knee replacement surgery. The
> success of the procedure is predicated on understanding the patient's
> clinical and radiographic presentation and proper preoperative assess-
> ment and planning.

> Talar dome lesions (TDL) have increasingly been the focus of interest of
> many foot and ankle surgeons over the past decade. The most important
> treatment aspect of TDL is diagnosis, so that appropriate treatment pro-
> tocols can be enacted in a timely and stepwise manner. Minor or mild
> TDL may be treated conservatively, while severe acute or chronic TDL
> can be addressed with various surgical interventions. By being aware of
> all practical treatment options and their indications, success rates, bene-
> fits, risks, and alternative options, specialists will be able to make an in-
> formed decision on appropriate care selection after perusing this article.

> Arthrosis of the ankle joint, typically posttraumatic in nature, can affect
> younger and older populations alike. A multitude of procedures exist for treat-
> ment, such as arthrodesis, total joint replacement, arthrodiastasis, and artic-
> ular repair. Current literature has demonstrated success in articular surface
> repair and arthrodiastasis as separate procedures. This article reviews the
> technique of ankle arthrodiastasis and interpositional ankle exostectomy,
> consisting of background, mechanism of action, indications, patient selec-
> tion criteria, complications, and advantages in the current literature.

> Ankle joint arthrodesis should be considered the gold standard procedure
> for end-stage ankle arthritis in the appropriate patient. Incisional approach

and fixation technique should be based on the patient and specific needs. Arthrodesis can be achieved with adequate resection of cartilage, good compression across the fusion site, stable fixation, proper postoperative protocol, and patient compliance. It is important to remember that positioning of the ankle joint is a keystone in ankle arthrodesis. There are complications that can arise from the ankle fusion, including the need for further surgical intervention owing to arthritis in the subtalar and midtarsal joints.

Combined arthrodesis of the ankle and subtalar joint is a challenging but potentially rewarding procedure for certain patients. The author discusses multiple aspects of the procedure from patient counseling to postoperative complications.

In the early 1970s, total ankle replacement was criticized because of poor outcomes with initial implant designs. Modifications were made that lead to the development of several generations of implants. The early shortcomings gave researchers and surgeons the impetus to improve implant designs and surgical technique. Total ankle replacement has become more widely accepted in recent years because of improved design and survivorship rates for the implants, as well as improved patient satisfaction scores. Indications for total ankle replacement have broadened. To continue these successes, it is important for surgeons to select appropriate patients for this procedure.

Total ankle joint replacement (TAR) has been offered as an alternative to ankle joint arthrodesis since the 1970s. TAR offers the benefit of perseveration of joint motion, with potential decreased occurrence of adjacent joint degeneration, and a more expedient path to weight bearing. Since their introduction, TAR devices have undergone a variety of modifications, specifically in regards to the number and type of components used.

Skin grafting provides an efficient way for diabetic wound closure when standard conservative therapy has failed and primary surgical closure is not an option. Pinch grafting provides an alternate method that can provide durable closure for soft tissue loss in the diabetic foot. An overview of this technique and its indications for diabetic foot wounds is presented.

An Overview of Bone Grafting Techniques for the Diabetic Charcot Foot and Ankle

Crystal L. Ramanujam, Zacharia Facaros, and Thomas Zgonis

Surgical options for diabetic Charcot neuroarthropathy of the foot and ankle must take into consideration the challenging environment for bone healing that accompanies these complex pathologic conditions. Bone grafting has established an important role in reconstructive surgery to promote bone formation, replacement, and repair. This article provides an overview of available bone grafting methods in conjunction with a review of the literature on these techniques as they pertain to diabetic Charcot foot and ankle reconstruction.

CLINICS IN PODIATRIC MEDICINE AND SURGERY

FORTHCOMING ISSUES

January 2013
Primary Total Ankle Replacement
Thomas S. Roukis, DPM, *Guest Editor*

April 2013
Revision Total Ankle Replacement
Thomas S. Roukis, DPM, *Guest Editor*

July 2013
Advances in Forefoot Surgery
Charles Zelen, DPM, *Guest Editor*

RECENT ISSUES

July 2012
Contemporary Controversies in Foot & Ankle Surgery
Neal M. Blitz, DPM, *Guest Editor*

April 2012
Foot and Ankle Trauma
Denise Mandi, DPM, *Guest Editor*

January 2012
Arthrodesis of the Foot and Ankle
Steven F. Boc, DPM and
Vincent Muscarella, DPM, *Guest Editors*

Foreword
Ankle Arthritis

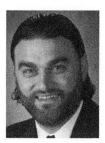

Thomas Zgonis, DPM, FACFAS
Consulting Editor

This edition of *Clinics in Podiatric Medicine and Surgery* focuses on the conservative and surgical treatment of ankle arthritis. Procedures including primary and revisional ankle arthrodesis, ankle arthroplasty, ankle arthrodiastasis, as well as correctional osteotomies to address the arthritic ankle are well covered by the invited authors with personal experience in this pathology. A review and treatment of talar osteochondral lesions are also presented in detail. Posttraumatic ankle arthritis is a common pathology and outcomes can vary according to the severity of the initial injury as well as the patient's activity level and comorbidities.

The guest editor, Dr Burks, and his colleagues were chosen for their surgical expertise in the treatment of ankle arthritis. I am thankful for their significant contributions to and support of the *Clinics in Podiatric Medicine and Surgery.*

Thomas Zgonis, DPM, FACFAS
Division of Podiatric Medicine and Surgery
Department of Orthopaedic Surgery
University of Texas Health Science Center San Antonio
7703 Floyd Curl Drive–MSC 7776
San Antonio, TX 78229, USA

E-mail address:
zgonis@uthscsa.edu

Clin Podiatr Med Surg 29 (2012) xi
http://dx.doi.org/10.1016/j.cpm.2012.08.012   **podiatric.theclinics.com**
0891-8422/12/$ – see front matter © 2012 Elsevier Inc. All rights reserved.

Preface

Ankle Arthritis

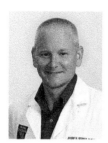

Jesse B. Burks, DPM, MS, FACFAS
Guest Editor

Degeneration of any joint can be a life-changing and disabling condition for a large segment of the population. Regardless of the cause, progressive loss of the articular surface and the management of the associated pain can be a challenge to any physician or surgeon—in any specialty. The ankle, because of its small surface area and high weight-bearing demands, can be especially difficult to manage conservatively and can also pose problems surgically for the same reasons. Even in cases where there are no other complicating factors—such as tibial or hindfoot malalignment—it can be difficult to reduce pain and restore even a remote semblance of normal gait.

I would like to thank all of my authors who contributed. Ankle arthritis is a very broad topic and I think the contributors have done an excellent job of both reviewing pertinent literature and adding their own personal clinical insights and experience. I am sure that making the time to contribute to this edition was challenging for them all, but I feel they have done an exceptional job of meeting that challenge.

Jesse B. Burks, DPM, MS, FACFAS
OrthoSurgeons
#5 St. Vincent Circle, Suite 410
Little Rock, AR 72205, USA

E-mail address:
jesse.burks@orthosurgeons.com

Clin Podiatr Med Surg 29 (2012) xiii
http://dx.doi.org/10.1016/j.cpm.2012.08.010
podiatric.theclinics.com

Supramalleolar Osteotomy for Realignment of the Ankle Joint

Noman A. Siddiqui, DPM, MHA, AACFAS*, John E. Herzenberg, MD,
Bradley M. Lamm, DPM

KEYWORDS

- Supramalleolar osteotomy • Focal dome osteotomy • Ankle deformity
- Deformity planning • Ankle Arthritis • Ankle realignment • Ankle malalignment
- Distal tibial ostetotomy

KEY POINTS

- Supramalleolar osteotomy is an extraarticular procedure that realigns the mechanical axis, thereby restoring ankle function.
- The literature discussing knee arthritis has shown that realignment osteotomies of the tibia improve function and prolong total knee replacement surgery.
- The success of the procedure is predicated on understanding the patient's clinical and radiographic presentation and proper preoperative assessment and planning.

INTRODUCTION

Distal tibia and ankle deformities are complex because rarely are these deformities uniplanar and without sequelae. These deformities are challenging and can lead to impaired ankle/foot mechanics, which result in osteoarthritis, pain, and dysfunction. Supramalleloar osteotomy of the distal tibia is used to realign the ankle and foot to the leg, thus improving function while preserving articular integrity of the ankle and relieving pain.[1-3] Supramalleolar osteotomy is an extraarticular procedure that realigns the mechanical axis, thereby restoring ankle function.[1,4] The procedure is versatile and can address uniplanar and oblique plane deformities due to osteoarthritis, malunited ankle/pilon fractures, malunited ankle fusions, and congenital and developmental deformities.[1-3,5-9] This osteotomy can address ankle procurvatum/recurvatum, varus/valgus, internal/external rotation, equinus, calcaneus, and limb length discrepancy. Clinical and radiographic preoperative planning is critical to identify the level

International Center for Limb Lenghtening/Rubin Institute for Advanced Orthopedics, Sinai Hospital of Baltimore, 2401 W. Belvedere Avenue, Baltimore MD 21215, USA
* Corresponding author.
E-mail address: nsiddiqu@lifebridgehealth.org

Clin Podiatr Med Surg 29 (2012) 465–482
http://dx.doi.org/10.1016/j.cpm.2012.07.002   **podiatric.theclinics.com**

and magnitude of deformity. The goal of this article is to outline the indications/contra-indications, clinical evaluation, radiographic preoperative planning, surgical technique, and postoperative care.

Indications for Supramalleolar Osteotomies

Supramalleolar osteotomies may be indicated for the following problems:

- Osteoarthritis
- Malunited distal tibia fractures
- Malaligned ankle fusions
- Congenital and developmental deformities[1,3,6,8,10–13]

Various factors can result in disability from the deformities mentioned, and understanding the pathomechanics of each will assist the surgeon in preservation of the ankle mortise.

OSTEOARTHRITIS

Osteoarthritis of the ankle has been shown to occur from malalignment of the ankle joint.[1,2,4–6,14] Malalignment results in uneven distribution of forces, which can lead to early wear of the articular surface and degenerative changes in the ankle.[1,15] Ramsey and Hamilton[16] in their posttraumatic ankle fracture experiments concluded that lateral talar displacement by 1 mm reduces the tibiotalar contact area by 42%. Similarly, Tarr and colleagues[21] reported further evidence of the effects of malalignment of the distal tibia and decrease in tibiotalar contact. Other factors such as inadequate subtalar joint inversion/eversion, ligamentous laxity, and muscle imbalance can further contribute to unequal loading of the ground reaction forces about the ankle joint. Supramalleolar osteotomy will realign the malaligned ankle joint, thus equally distributing the forces on the joint. Realignment, through osteotomy, improves ankle joint mechanics and slows the progression of osteoarthritis.

In cases of severe osteoarthritis with a concomitant malalignment of the ankle or distal tibia, salvage of the ankle may not be possible with supramalleolar osteotomy alone. In such instances, supramalleolar realignment followed by total ankle replacement has been reported in the literature.[17,18] Also, for ankle joint preservation, a supramalleolar osteotomy followed by hinged external fixation ankle distraction has been reported.[19,20]

MALUNITED DISTAL TIBIA

Malunions of the distal tibia are common complications of traumatic injury. These deformities make ambulation difficult and frequently require surgical intervention. Deformities greater then 15° in the distal tibia can decrease the tibiotalar contact area by 42%.[21] Unequal forces on the mortise result in pain and advance the deterioration of the ankle joint. Malunions can occur in the sagittal, frontal, transverse, or oblique plane and increase abnormal loading on the ankle joint and the lower extremity.[1]

SAGITTAL PLANE DEFORMITY

Procurvatum or recurvatum deformity occurs in the sagittal plane and is best visualized on a standing lateral radiograph (**Fig.** 1A–D). Compensation for the deformity is by ankle joint plantar flexion or dorsiflexion. Because there is less ankle joint dorsiflexion available, procurvatum deformities are not tolerated as well as recurvatum

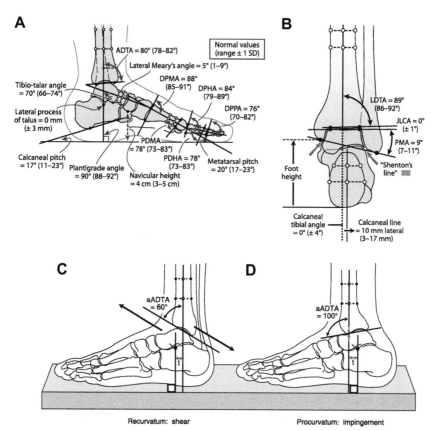

Fig. 1. Normal angles of the foot. (*A*) Normal lateral radiograph angles. (*B*) Normal anterior-posterior radiograph angles. (*C*) Recurvatum increases shear forces of the distal tibia and displaces the foot anteriorly and increases the lever arm of the foot, making ambulation difficult. (*D*) Procurvatum creates anterior ankle impingement due to decrease in ankle joint dorsiflexion. Procurvatum is less tolerated then recurvatum deformity. (*Reprinted from* Paley D. Ankle and foot considerations. In: Herzenberg JE, editor. Principles of deformity correction. Springer Verlag; 2002. p. 571–645, with permission; and Copyright 2011, Rubin Institute for Advanced Orthopedics, Sinai Hospital of Baltimore.)

deformities. Patients with procurvatum also complain of ankle joint impingement because of limited ankle joint dorsiflexion, whereas those with recurvatum have less plantar flexor strength at push off. This foot position does not maximize the arc of motion within the ankle and creates unequal load on the articular surfaces. When revising this malposition, it is necessary to convert the motion that is present into a more functional arc. Soft tissue contractures of the ankle and subtalar capsule, along with a tight heel cord may need to be addressed. The release of these structures assists in improving the motion of the foot and ankle. The compensatory soft tissue contractures are discussed in greater detail later in this article.

One must maintain axial alignment in the sagittal plane. Anterior or posterior translation of the foot with respect to the distal tibia, such that the middiaphyseal line of the tibia passes through the lateral process of the talus, allows the foot to function anatomically (see **Fig. 1**A–D). When this line is posterior to the lateral process of the talus, the foot becomes longer, thus increasing the lever arm on the foot, making walking more difficult.

FRONTAL PLANE DEFORMITY

A frontal plane deformity is characterized by varus or valgus malunions of the ankle or distal tibia. Malalignment in the frontal plane of the ankle joint is best evaluated on a standing anterior-posterior radiograph. Normally, varus malalignment does not result in degeneration of the ankle joint because of the buttressing effect of the medial malleolus. The wide medial malleolus and the medial talar facet articulation serve to maintain the contact area and the dispersion of forces between the tibia and talus (**Fig. 2**A). However, varus malalignment does create problems in the subtalar joint and first ray, which can become symptomatic and painful. Normally, the subtalar joint compensates for varus malalignment of the ankle through subtalar eversion. However, if compensatory subtalar joint motion is not present, the forefoot compensates by plantarflexing the first ray. The plantar flexion of the first ray increases the arch and decreases the weightbearing surface area of the foot.[1]

The valgus ankle leads to degeneration of the ankle joint (see **Fig. 2**B). During normal single leg stance, the ground reaction force vector passes lateral to the ankle and subtalar joint and imparts a valgus thrust on those joints. In a valgus ankle, there is increased load on the lateral tibiotalar surfaces because of increased lateralization of the ground reaction vector (GRV). Chronic loading of the ankle in this manner can disrupt the tibial-fibular articulation and lead to disruption of the syndesmosis, lateral translation of the talus in the ankle mortise, and degeneration of the articular surfaces of the tibia and talus.

MALUNITED FUSION

Similar to a malaligned ankle joint, a malunited ankle fusion can also create painful ambulation for the joints proximal and distal to the fusion mass. The advantage of

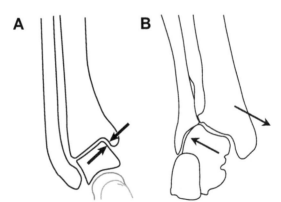

Fig. 2. Varus and valgus ankle deformity. (*A*) In varus deformities, the medial malleolus buttresses the medial talar facet and maintain tibiotalar contact area, thus decreasing risk of osteoarthritis. (*B*) Ankle valgus deformity leads to unequal tibiotalar contact and progresses to osteoarthritis more rapidly because of lateralization of the ground reaction vector. (*Reprinted from* Paley D. Ankle and foot considerations. In: Herzenberg JE, editor. Principles of deformity correction. Springer Verlag; 2002. p. 571–645; with permission.)

performing realignment osteotomies, in instances of prior fusion, is that they can be performed into the fusion mass, without fear of violating the articular surface. If there is an associated limb length discrepancy, one can lengthen the limb simultaneously using the same osteotomy, with the use of external fixation. In certain instances, soft tissue integrity can limit correction through a previous incision or osteotomy because of previous or multiple surgeries. Supramalleolar osteotomies can provide an alternative zone of correction in deformity repair. In populations with malunited fusions, there are multiple adjacent joint compensatory mechanisms that must be considered. Compensation is discussed later in this article.

CONGENITAL AND DEVELOPMENTAL DEFORMITIES

Congenital and developmental deformities, such as clubfoot, cerebral palsy, fibular hemimelia, Charcot-Marie-Tooth, myelomeningocele, amongst others can cause deformity that is resistant to correction. These deformities can significantly affect the ankle joint complex. Supramalleolar osteotomy has been used successfully to treat resistant congenital deformities[22,23] and aims to realign the foot to the leg and create a plantigrade foot.

INTERNAL/EXTERNAL ROTATION

Tibial torsion deformities are most common in childhood and normally resolve spontaneously.[23] Symptomatic medial and lateral torsion deformities that do not resolve by 8 years of age may require tibial derotation osteotomy. The osteotomy to correct rotational deformity is made in the distal tibial metaphysis. After correction is achieved, fixation with smooth Steinman pins protects the physis. Typically, only severe or symptomatic rotational deformities are addressed with a supramalleolar osteotomy. However, rotational deformities that are present in combination with osseous malalignment are addressed simultaneously in the distal tibia.

CONTRAINDICATIONS

Relative contraindications for supramalleolar osteotomy include the following:

- Nonambulatory status
- Impaired vascular status
- Presence of soft tissue or bony infection
- Distal tibial nonunion that has not been addressed

CLINICAL PRESENTATION

A comprehensive history and physical examination is essential before proceeding with any intervention. The cause and effect of malalignment of the distal tibia must be identified. For example, when working up a posttraumatic deformity, knowing the type of injury (bony and/or soft tissue, high vs low energy, open or closed, intraarticular vs extraarticular), subsequent management, and compensatory deformity assist in preoperative planning. Examination of the patient's shoes may reveal a deformity specific wear pattern and/or shoe modification.

During the physical examination, it is important to note painful areas of the foot and ankle. Supramalleolar deformities can occur at the level of the ankle or juxta-articular, which may induce ankle instability. In such cases, a clinical stress of the ankle (talar tilt and anterior draw) should be performed. Ankle varus deformity is tolerated less well when there is adequate subtalar joint motion because the subtalar joint generally has less eversion compensation available than inversion (**Fig. 3**A).[1] However, in ankle

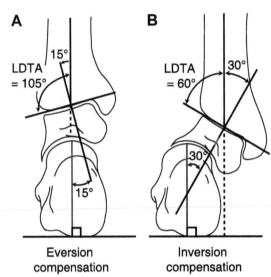

Fig. 3. Compensation for ankle varus or valgus. (*A*) Ankle varus is compensated by subtalar joint eversion. In this figure, a 15° ankle varus is compensated by 15° of subtalar joint eversion. (*B*) Ankle valgus is compensated well because of the greater inversion available at the subtalar joint. A 30° ankle valgus will compensate by subtalar joint inversion of 30°. (*Reprinted from* Paley D. Ankle and foot considerations. In: Herzenberg JE, editor. Principles of deformity correction. Springer Verlag; 2002. p. 571–645; with permission.)

varus deformity, lateral column pain due to subfibular impingement is a common physical examination finding and may require additional osseous procedures.[4] Ankle valgus deformities are tolerated well because there is greater inversion compensation available at the subtalar joint (see **Fig. 3**B).[1,24] However, these patients may complain of pain at the subtalar joint or develop first ray symptoms if compensation is not available. The compensatory mechanisms of the foot, as they relate to various ankle deformities, are discussed later in greater detail.

Muscle and tendon contracture should be assessed during the clinical examination. Ankle deformity can cause a fallen arch, leading to arch pain, which may be attributed to posterior tibial tendon tendonitis. If the ankle deformity is long standing, the tendon will ultimately fail and will require repair or transfer augmentation. Equinus evaluation is critical in addressing the deformity. A Silfverskiöld test of the ankle joint with the knee extended and flexed determines relative tightness of the gastrocnemius and soleus muscles. Any bony impingement or crepitus will also be noted with range of motion evaluation of the ankle, subtalar, midtarsal, and digital joints. Any bony impingement or crepitus will also be noted with range of motion evaluation of ankle, subtalar, midtarsal, and digital joints. Any bony impingement or crepitus will also be noted with range of motion evaluation of ankle, subtalar, midtarsal, and digital joints. Previous injury or surgery can lead to areas of poor circulation or sensation. Therefore, it is necessary to assess adequate vascular status, and note any neurological deficits prior to surgery.

Weightbearing examination is done to evaluate the compensated pedal position in the face of an ankle deformity. Axial evaluation of the heel-leg relationship from behind the patient is critical. Also, sagittal and transverse plane weightbearing pedal assessment is important. Finally, rotation malalignment should be documented by placing the patient prone to measure the thigh-foot angle. Gait analysis provides further insight into the effects of the deformity on ambulation.

RADIOGRAPHIC PLANNING

Radiographs are the building blocks for preoperative planning for the supramalleolar osteotomy. Multiplanar radiographs are obtained and assessed for angular and translational relationships by drawing planning lines, angles, and reference points. This deformity analysis allows for identification of the level and magnitude of the deformity. Standard lower limb reference points and measurements for consideration should be done before any surgical realignment (see **Figs. 1** and **4**).[1,24]

On a lateral radiograph of the ankle to include the tibia, the anatomic posterior proximal tibial angle is the relationship between the tibial middiaphyseal line and the articular surface of the proximal tibia (normal, 77°–84°). The anatomic anterior distal tibial angle (ADTA) is the angular relationship between the tibial middiaphyseal line and the tibial plafond (normal, 78°–82°). The lateral process of the talus, which also serves as the center of ankle joint range of motion, should fall on the tibial middiaphyseal line. Anterior or posterior displacement is not considered anatomic.

On an anterior posterior radiograph of the ankle to include the tibia, the anatomic medial proximal tibial angle is the relationship between the tibial middiaphyseal line and the articular surface of the proximal tibia (normal, 85°–90°). The anatomic lateral distal tibial angle is the angular relationship between the tibial middiaphyseal line and the tibial plafond (normal, 86°–92°). The center of the talar dome is located at the bisection between the medial and lateral aspects of the trochlea of the talus. The center of the talar dome is slightly lateral with respect to the tibial middiaphyseal line; deviation from this is not considered anatomic.

Frontal plane radiographs exhibit the calcaneus to tibial relationship. On a weightbearing long leg calcaneal axial and hindfoot alignment radiographs, the tibial middiaphyseal line should parallel the calcaneal bisection line (a parallel heel-to-leg relationship). Angulations greater or less than 0° to 2° of valgus are not considered anatomic.[24] On the hindfoot alignment view, the normal heel bisection is 5 to 10 mm lateral to the tibial middiaphyseal line.[25] Preoperative frontal plane relationships are helpful to distinguish malalignments between the ankle joint, subtalar joint, and calcaneus. A subtalar joint deformity is seen on the long leg calcaneal axial view, and an osseous calcaneal tuber deformity is visualized on the hindfoot alignment view. The hindfoot alignment

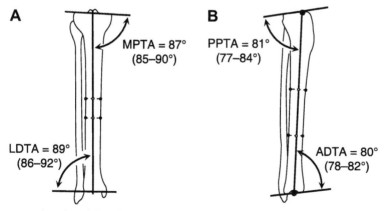

Fig. 4. Normal angles of the tibia. (*A*) Normal anterior-posterior radiograph tibial alignment and joint orientation angles. (*B*) Normal lateral radiograph tibial alignment and joint orientation angles. (*Reprinted from* Paley D. Ankle and foot considerations. In: Herzenberg JE, editor. Principles of deformity correction. Springer Verlag; 2002. p. 571–645; with permission.)

or "Saltzman" view allows for visualization of the ankle joint and the angular measurement of the middiaphyseal line of the tibia to the calcaneal bisection.[25] Therefore, both frontal plane radiographs are critical to appropriately assess the preoperative alignment/relationship between the talus, tibia, and calcaneus.

On the anterior-posterior view of the ankle, one must include the tibia to thoroughly assess the deformity. Subtle deformity in the proximal tibia leads to severe malalignment at the ankle level. However, the closer the deformity to the ankle joint, the greater the effect on the ankle. For example, a 10° varus deformity in the proximal tibia distorts the lower extremity mechanical axis significantly as compared with a 10° varus deformity in the distal tibia.

Measuring the ADTA on the lateral radiograph distinguishes the degree of procurvatum or recurvatum deformity of the distal tibia. The stress maximum dorsiflexion lateral radiograph also allows evaluation of equinus. Other radiographic findings on the anterior-posterior and lateral radiographs that are useful in preoperative planning are the evaluation of the articular surface, loose joint bodies, osteophytes, nonunions, bony defects, and infected sequestra. If the possibility of a nonunion is present from a prior injury or surgery, a preoperative computed tomography scan can characterize and eliminate the geometry of the nonunion.

COMPENSATION

Distal tibial deformities lead to compensatory motion at adjacent joints. Combining the radiographic and clinical presentation will give the surgeon a greater understanding of the deformity and how the patient can or cannot compensate for their deformity. In the frontal plane, the subtalar joint provides for 20° to 30° of inversion and 10° to 15° of eversion.[1,24] If a deformity is greater than the available subtalar joint motion, additional compensation is accomplished by pronation and supination of the forefoot.[24] Therefore, the greater the mobility of the subtalar joint and forefoot, the greater the compensation for the tibia deformity (see **Fig. 3**A, B).

FRONTAL PLANE COMPENSATION

In the frontal plane, valgus deformity of the distal tibia is tolerated better than varus deformity because of the greater amount of subtalar joint motion that is available.[1,24] Distal tibial varus or valgus deformities that exceed the amount of compensation that is available result in compensatory forefoot supination and pronation. In cases of distal tibial varus that does not have adequate subtalar joint compensation, the first ray must compensate to bring the forefoot to the ground. The increased plantar flexion of the first ray increases arch height, thus decreasing the weightbearing surface of the foot. In instances of distal tibial valgus with inadequate subtalar joint inversion compensation, the forefoot supinates and the first ray dorsiflexes, thus resulting in a flattening of the arch and increasing the weightbearing surface of the foot.

Varus and valgus deformity of the distal tibia also move the GRV medial or lateral to the foot.[1,24] In normal gait, the GRV passes lateral to the ankle joint and imparts a valgus moment arm on the ankle joint. A valgus deformity further increases the load on the lateral aspect of the ankle joint and shift the talus further into the syndesmosis, which results in articular destruction. This deformity is common sequelae of an ankle fracture that has a shortened fibular or valgus tilt because of incomplete reduction. Varus deformity of the distal tibia or ankle moves the GRV medially; however, this is not likely to result in degenerative changes. The broader medial malleolus articular surface offloads the increase in pressure and spares the ankle from degenerative changes. However, it is more symptomatic because the subtalar joint cannot compensate as much in eversion as it can in inversion. Thus, there are increased likelihood of subtalar arthritis and painful forefoot symptoms in a patient.

SAGITTAL PLANE COMPENSATION

In the sagittal plane, the foot compensates for procurvatum or recurvatum deformity of the distal tibia, respectively, by ankle joint dorsiflexion or plantar flexion.[24] Normal ankle joint range of motion is 50° of plantar flexion and 20° of dorsiflexion. Because there is greater plantar flexion available, the foot compensates for recurvatum quite well. However, distal tibial recurvatum is more joint destructive because the articular surface is not as covered and tilts it anteriorly, and because of this, it is not painful early on and is typically recognized after the condition has severely progressed. Recurvatum of the distal tibia is also compensated for by the triceps surae. Recurvatum of the distal tibia displaces the center of rotation of the ankle joint anteriorly, thus increasing the anterior lever arm. The triceps surae counter these forces by placing the foot in equinus and decreasing the plantar flexor push off the foot. Distal tibial procurvatum is typically more painful because it has limited compensation available through the ankle joint and results in anterior ankle joint impingement.[1,24] However, in procurvatum, the articular surface of the ankle joint is well covered in the mortise and is normally spared from deterioration.[1]

If the osseous deformity of the distal tibia is present for many years, the foot and ankle develop fixed compensatory compensation.[24] This fixed compensation is unmasked by correcting the deformity of the distal tibia. For example, correcting a distal tibial varus deformity via supramalleolar osteotomy can leave the foot in a valgus position, which is a result of unmasking a fixed subtalar eversion contracture.[24] Thus, one must identify the fixed compensatory position before proceeding with osseous correction of any deformity. This is accomplished by placing the foot in a position of maximum deformity. If it cannot reach the maximum deformity position, then a fixed compensatory contracture is present.[24] In the case of the distal tibial valgus with fixed compensatory subtalar varus contracture, the subtalar joint deformity must be addressed when performing supramalleolar corrective osteotomy.

TECHNIQUE

There are certain considerations when performing supramalleolar osteotomies. When soft tissue and bony considerations are of little concern, the osteotomy should be based primarily on the level or location of the apex of the deformity known as the center of rotation of angulation (CORA).[1] Using osteotomy principles, one can plan for proper realignment of the bony segments when performing osteotomy, at or away from the CORA.

When a corrective osteotomy is performed at the level of the CORA, the deformity is corrected by angulation alone. If the osteotomy is made a distance away from the CORA, compensatory translation must be achieved. The surgeon must be aware of bony and soft tissue considerations when performing correction to make the mechanical axis, after correction, collinear. For example, when correcting a procurvatum deformity with a CORA at the ankle joint, an anterior closing wedge osteotomy in the distal tibia will translate the foot anterior. If this is not accounted for, it will increase the lever arm or length of the foot, thus making ambulation more difficult.

In the frontal plane, this is best visualized in a distal tibial varus deformity by performing a closing wedge osteotomy of the distal tibia, with the CORA at the ankle joint. By removing the laterally based wedge, the tibial plafond can be translated laterally with respect to the mechanical axis of the tibia. Thus, to realign the axis, the distal fragment must be translated medially.

Another consideration is the level of the osteotomy. Supramalleloar osteotomies are most commonly performed in the excellent healing metaphyseal zone of the distal tibia. However, an osteotomy made in the diaphysis of the distal tibial (approximately 2.5 cm or proximal from the ankle joint) can lead to delayed healing. Cutting bone with an osteotome (low-energy osteotomy) is more likely to heal faster than with a power saw (high-energy osteotomy), which creates thermal necrosis. Soft tissue considerations are also important when performing supramalleolar osteotomy. When correcting deformities in the sagittal or frontal plane, one must be aware of the stretch or entrapment that is placed on the posterior tibial nerve. A correction of as little as 5° can cause the patient severe pain and discomfort.[19,20,26] A prophylactic tarsal tunnel release should be considered when planning for deformity correction.[26]

OPENING AND CLOSING WEDGE OSTEOTOMY

Wedge osteotomies are made for sagittal, frontal, or oblique plane deformities of the distal tibia. Planning for the deformity is made on the anterior-posterior and lateral radiographs of the ankle to include the tibia. In the frontal plane, a lateral distal tibial angle that is greater than 92° would indicate a varus deformity, whereas less than 86° indicates valgus deformity (see **Fig. 1**B). In the sagittal plane, when the ADTA is greater than 82°, a procurvatum deformity exists. Angulations less than 78° signify recurvatum (see **Fig. 1**A). A weightbearing erect leg radiograph (anterior-posterior view of the pelvis, femurs, tibias) allows accurate limb length measurements for preoperative planning. When length is needed, an acute opening wedge osteotomy with internal fixation or gradual opening wedge osteotomy with external fixation is performed, and when limb length equalization is not needed, an acute closing wedge osteotomy is used (**Fig. 5**).

The patient is placed on the table in a supine position under general or spinal/epidural anesthesia with a bump under the ipsilateral hip. A thigh tourniquet is used based on the surgeon's preference. The extremity is prepped above the level of the knee, such that the foot and knee alignment can be visualized. If deemed necessary (acute corrections greater than 10°, gradual corrections greater than 25°, deformity correction with lengthening, or prior scarring), the tarsal tunnel release is performed prophylactically before any osteotomy.[26] Under fluoroscopic guidance, the level of the osteotomy and the ankle joint are marked (**Fig. 6**).

An anterior ankle approach is made for sagittal plane deformities and either a lateral or a medial ankle incision is made for frontal plane deformities. Dissection is kept to a minimum while protection of the neurovascular bundle is used. When necessary, the incision is extended to the level of the ankle joint to excise any synovial capsule or osteophytic debris about the ankle joint or for repair of an osteochondral defect. Fluoroscopy is used to confirm complete ankle osteophyte resection. Also, fluoroscopic guidance is used to obtain the anterior-posterior and lateral distal tibia images to identify the level of the CORA. A 1.8-mm wire is inserted to mark the location of the CORA. Minimal periosteal dissection is performed to prepare for the osteotomy. A wedge osteotomy is typically performed using an intraoperative wire guidance technique; 1.8-mm Ilizarov wires are placed parallel to the ankle joint and perpendicular to the mechanical axis of the tibia. The wires meet at the apex or CORA of the deformity and are used as a guide for the wedge resection osteotomies. A wide oscillating saw is used to perform the cuts along each wire, either maintaining the far cortex or creating a through and through osteotomy. The far cortex serves as a hinge for the

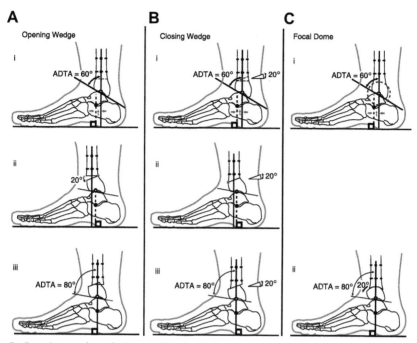

Fig. 5. Opening wedge, closing wedge, focal dome osteotomy. (*A*) (i) An ankle with recurvatum deformity is corrected with an opening wedge osteotomy. (ii) Note the posterior displacement of the foot after correction. (iii) The foot must be translated anteriorly to maintain anatomic alignment. (*B*) (i) A closing wedge osteotomy for the same deformity. (ii) The deformity correction realigns the anatomic ankle relationship but displaces the foot posteriorly. (iii) The foot is translated anterior to maintain anatomic alignment. (*C*) (i) Focal dome osteotomy is performed to correct the recurvatum deformity. (ii) Correction of the focal dome osteotomy is based around the CORA, thus positioning the foot into anatomic alignment without translation. (*Reprinted from* Paley D. Ankle and foot considerations. In: Herzenberg JE, editor. Principles of deformity correction. Springer Verlag; 2002. p. 571–645; with permission.)

opening wedge. The malalignment is reduced under fluoroscopic guidance and fixated. When an opening wedge osteotomy is performed, the defect is filled with bone graft and secured with internal fixation (plates, screws, pins). A closing wedge is performed and secured with internal fixation (plates, screws, pins, staples). A drain is typically placed, and the skin is closed in layers. Ideally, the supramalleolar osteotomy is performed in the metaphyseal bone. However, it is important to remember that an osteotomy away from the CORA will require secondary translation to realign the mechanical axis. In those instances, the osteotomy will be through and through and not hinged.

Beyond identifying the CORA and the magnitude of deformity, it is important to measure the length of the malleoli. When the tibia and fibula are not of equal deformity, then critical analysis of the plafond malleolar ankle (normal = 9°) is performed on an anterior-posterior radiograph of the ankle to include tibia. If the plafond malleolar angle is abnormal, then the tibia or fibula length differential must be measured. Based on this length, the surgeon will decide whether an acute of gradual correction is required to equalize the malleoli and restore balance to the mortise.

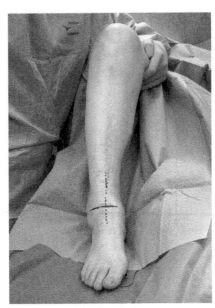

Fig. 6. Preoperative planning. The level of the ankle joint and incision is marked on the patient. (Copyright 2011, Rubin Institute for Advanced Orthopedics, Sinai Hospital of Baltimore.)

FOCAL DOME OSTEOTOMY

Focal dome osteotomies are used when the CORA is at the level of the ankle joint and are performed open or percutaneous.[1,27,28] In the frontal or sagittal plane, a percutaneous 3-stab incision from the anterior or medial approach, respectively or an open incision is used.

When performing a focal dome osteotomy, a tibial half pin a few millimeters above the ankle joint is placed. The half pin must be parallel to the ankle joint in the frontal and sagittal planes, which is confirmed on fluoroscopy (**Fig. 7**). A focal dome osteotomy guide or Rancho Cube (Smith and Nephew, Memphis, TN) is used to guide multiple drill holes along the osteotomy in a domelike fashion such that it is completed through the medial and lateral cortices of the metaphysis of the tibia (**Fig. 8**).

When performing a percutaneous supramalleolar osteotomy, multiple stab incisions are carefully placed to avoid the neurovascular bundle. Osteotomies are placed through the incisions, and the multiple drill holes are connected to complete the through and through osteotomy and confirmed under fluoroscopic guidance. A fibular osteotomy is also performed distal or at the level of the tibial osteotomy by making a small stab incision and using multiple drill holes via a 1.8-mm Ilizarov wire. The holes are connected with a small Hoke osteotome, and a through and through osteotomy is made, which is confirmed on fluoroscopy. The osteotome is rotated to help rotate the osteotomy fragment. The deformity is reduced and fixated with internal or external fixation. Final radiographs are used to confirm the reduced alignment and correction of the mechanical axis (**Fig. 9**). A medium hemovac drain is placed, and wound closure is performed in layers. The patient is placed in a splint or bivalved cast when internal fixation is used and admitted to the hospital for pain and drain management.

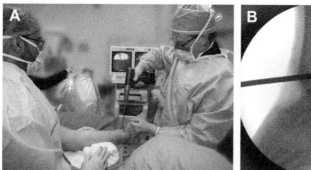
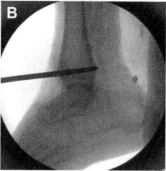

Fig. 7. Intraoperative views. (*A*) The half pin is predrilled carefully into the distal tibia with a tissue protector sleeve at the CORA of the deformity. (*B*) A half pin is placed perpendicular to the anatomic axis of the tibia. (Copyright 2011, Rubin Institute for Advanced Orthopedics, Sinai Hospital of Baltimore.)

GIGLI SAW OSTEOTOMY

An alternative method for supramalleolar osteotomy is the Gigli saw. This method is percutaneous and is used to make a complete osteotomy of either the tibia or fibula or both. Three small incisions are used, 2 medial and one lateral. The orientation of the medial incisions is transverse and the lateral incision is longitudinal. At the level of planned osteotomy site, a medial transverse incision is made just medial to the tibialis anterior tendon, and the periosteum on the anterior aspect of the tibia and fibula are elevated until the elevator tents the skin over the lateral fibula. A second transverse incision is made medially, just anterior to the tibialis posterior tendon. An elevator is used to raise the posterior periosteum of the tibia and fibula. A third, longitudinal fibular incision is then made where the elevator protrudes over the fibula. A long, curved hemostat is used to pass a heavy suture from medial to lateral. The suture is then tied to the Gigli saw and carefully pulled from the medial to lateral incision. The suture

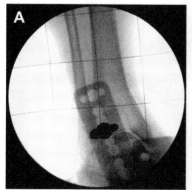
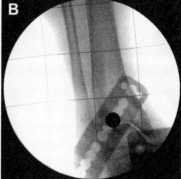

Fig. 8. Intraoperative view. (*A*) Using a focal dome osteotomy guide, the lateral and medial margin of the osteotomy on the tibia is confirmed. (*B*) The osteotomy should be performed in the metaphyseal bone of the distal tibia, no greater than approximately 2 cm above the ankle joint. (Copyright 2011, Rubin Institute for Advanced Orthopedics, Sinai Hospital of Baltimore.)

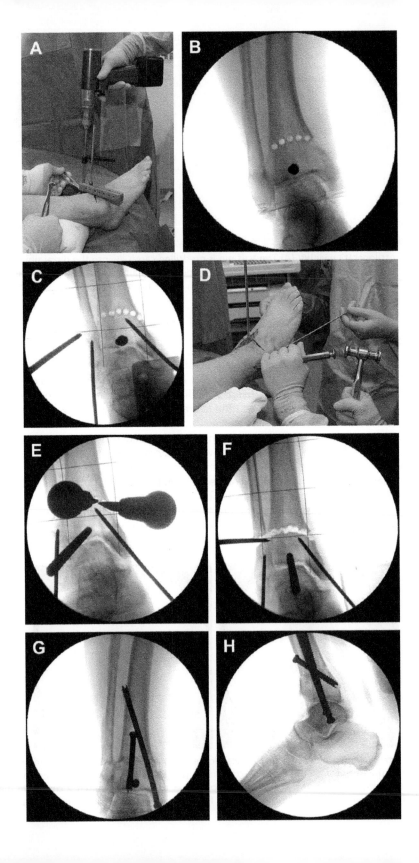

is then passed from the lateral incision to the posteromedial tibial third incision, which is transverse. The Gigli saw is then directed through the posteromedial tibial incision. Using a sawing motion, the tibia and fibula are cut from lateral to medial until the Gigli saw is close to completing the tibial cut. Small retractors protect skin and tendons. An elevator is placed between the soft tissue and medial tibial cortex to protect the saw from cutting the skin. The osteotomy is then completed; the Gigli saw is safely removed. The through and through cut is visualized under fluoroscopy. The realignment is now achieved and fixated with internal or external fixation. Typically, a Gigli saw osteotomy is performed for oblique plane deformities or deformities that require simultaneous lengthening.

Postoperatively, the patient is admitted for pain control and drain management. The patient is discharged non-weightbearing on crutches or walker with internal fixation and weightbearing as tolerated with external fixation. Consider prophylactic anticoagulation for deep vein thrombosis with low-molecular-weight heparin for 30 days in patients who have at least one risk factor for deep vein thrombosis.

FIXATION METHODS

There are various advantages and disadvantages of using internal or external fixation. The advantages of internal fixation are that (1) the hardware can be safely placed, (2) there are numerous options (plates, screws) available, and (3) there is surgeon comfort. The disadvantages of internal fixation are greater dissection and exposure, loss of purchase, hardware failure, and non-weightbearing cast immobilization osteoporosis. The advantages of external fixation are minimal dissection, early weightbearing, showering, correction of concomitant deformities (ie, equinus, limb length discrepancy), and avoidance of areas of infection or poor soft tissue. The disadvantages include pin site infections, patient fear and management, the need for a second surgery for removal, and that it is technically challenging to apply. The surgeon should choose the method that can accomplish the best result based on both the patient's condition and his or her experience and skill level (**Fig. 10**).

TOTAL ANKLE JOINT REPLACEMENTS

Coetzee[17] reported 50% failure of ankle replacement of patients with varus greater than 20°. Supramalleolar osteotomies may be combined with total ankle replacements either in a prior staged procedure or simultaneously.[10,18] As total ankle replacement designs improve and the durability of such implants is increased, they will become increasingly valuable as adjunct procedures with deformity correction of the distal tibia. The long-term follow-up of these procedures is still needed.

◀ ——————————————————————————

Fig. 9. Focal dome osteotomy. (A) The focal dome guide allows for precise drill-hole placement in an arc-like pattern. (B) Confirming the drill holes under fluoroscopy before completing the osteotomy. (C) The fibular osteotomy is performed through a small incision below the level of the multiple drill holes in the tibia. The guide pins for screw placement are accurately positioned before osteotomy completion. (D) The osteotome allows for a low-energy fibular osteotomy, which improves the healing potential after correction. (E) Multiple osteotomies are used to connect the tibial drill holes before a through and through osteotomy is completed. (F) Displacement of the tibia and fibula with an osteotome ensures the osteotomy is complete. (G) After osseous reduction, large cannulated screws are used to maintain the correction with the ankle mortise in anatomic alignment. (H) Lateral view confirms accurate alignment and screw placement. A large osteophyte was resected from the front of the joint. (Copyright 2011, Rubin Institute for Advanced Orthopedics, Sinai Hospital of Baltimore.)

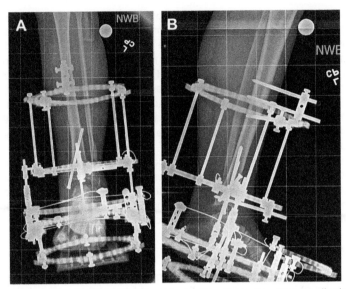

Fig. 10. Supramalleolar osteotomy with gradual ankle distraction. Supramalleolar osteotomies are combined with gradual ankle joint distraction to preserve the articular surface of the ankle. (*A*) Anterior-posterior radiographic view. (*B*) Lateral radiographic view. (Copyright 2011, Rubin Institute for Advanced Orthopedics, Sinai Hospital of Baltimore.)

SUMMARY

As discussed earlier, ankle malalignment can lead to wear and ankle arthritis. Recent attention has been given to quality of life of patients with end-stage hip and ankle arthritis. A study found that end-stage ankle arthritis resulted in mental and physical disability, which was as severe as end-stage hip arthritis.[29,30] This finding is significant given that fewer options are available to those with ankle arthritis than those with hip arthritis. Ankle replacement systems have not been as reliable as hip replacements in providing long-term relief of pain, increased motion, and return to full activity. Therefore, maintenance and restoration of an anatomic ankle joint is important in preserving a pain free range of motion. Hinterman and colleagues[30] performed a prospective study on 48 patients who underwent a supramalleolar osteotomy for malunited fractures of the ankle. In their study, 87.5% related good or excellent results after 7 years of follow-up and 91% had little to no progression of arthritis radiographically.

Supramalleloar osteotomy can address deformities of the distal tibia and ankle joint. They are challenging to perform accurately but restore normal mechanics of the foot and ankle. Restoration of normal mechanics ensures the equal distribution of functional forces on the joints of the foot and ankle, which in many cases will prevent or prolong the progression of end-stage ankle arthritis and allow for improved function. This osteotomy is analogous to corrective high tibial osteotomies performed in the proximal tibia to correct varus/valgus malalignment of the tibia. The literature discussing knee arthritis has shown that realignment osteotomies of the tibia improve function and prolong total knee replacement surgery.[31–34]

Supramalleolar osteotomy can be successful but requires a complete understanding of the deformity. Multiple methods to perform the osteotomy and fixate the correction are available. The success of the procedure is predicated on understanding the patient's clinical and radiographic presentation and proper preoperative assessment and planning.

REFERENCES

1. Paley D, Herzenberg JE, editors. Ankle and foot Considerations. Principles of Deformity Correction. Berlin: Springer-Verlag; 2002. p. 571–645.
2. Knupp M, Bolliger L, Hintermann B. Treatment of posttraumatic varus ankle deformity with supramalleolar osteotomy. Foot Ankle Clin 2012;17(1):95–102.
3. Horn DM, Fragomen AT, Rozbruch SR. Supramalleolar osteotomy using circular external fixation with six-axis deformity correction of the distal tibia. Foot Ankle Int 2011;32(10):986–93.
4. Lee WC, Moon JS, Lee HS, et al. Alignment of ankle and hindfoot in early stage ankle osteoarthritis. Foot Ankle Int 2011;32(7):693–9.
5. Paley D. The correction of complex foot deformities using Ilizarov's distraction osteotomies. Clin Orthop Relat Res 1993;(293):97–111.
6. Knupp M, Stufkens SA, Bolliger L, et al. Classification and treatment of supramalleolar deformities. Foot Ankle Int 2011;32(11):1023–31.
7. Knupp M, Stufkens SA, van Bergen CJ, et al. Effect of supramalleolar varus and valgus deformities on the tibiotalar joint: a cadaveric study. Foot Ankle Int 2011; 32(6):609–15.
8. Stamatis ED, Cooper PS, Myerson MS. Supramalleolar osteotomy for the treatment of distal tibial angular deformities and arthritis of the ankle joint. Foot Ankle Int 2003;24(10):754–64.
9. Stamatis ED, Myerson MS. Supramalleolar osteotomy: indications and technique [review]. Foot Ankle Clin 2003;8(2):317–33.
10. Ryssman D, Myerson MS. Surgical strategies: the management of varus ankle deformity with joint replacement. Foot Ankle Int 2011;32(2):217–24.
11. Lee KB, Cho YJ. Oblique supramalleolar opening wedge osteotomy without fibular osteotomy for varus deformity of the ankle. Foot Ankle Int 2009;30(6):565–7.
12. Harstall R, Lehmann O, Krause F, et al. Supramalleolar lateral closing wedge osteotomy for the treatment of varus ankle arthrosis. Foot Ankle Int 2007;28(5):542–8.
13. Sen C, Kocaoglu M, Eralp L, et al. Correction of ankle and hindfoot deformities by supramalleolar osteotomy. Foot Ankle Int 2003;24(1):22–8.
14. Heywood AW. Supramalleolar osteotomy in the management of the rheumatoid hindfoot. Clin Orthop Relat Res 1983;(177):76–81.
15. Yablon IG, Heller FG, Shouse L. The key role of the lateral malleolus in displaced fractures of the ankle. J Bone Joint Surg Am 1977;59(2):169–73.
16. Ramsey PL, Hamilton W. Changes in tibiotalar area of contact caused by lateral talar shift. J Bone Joint Surg Am 1976;58(3):356–7.
17. Coetzee JC. Management of varus or valgus ankle deformity with ankle replacement. Foot Ankle Clin 2008;13(3):509–20, x.
18. Tan KJ, Myerson MS. Planning correction of the varus ankle deformity with ankle replacement. Foot Ankle Clin 2012;17(1):103–15.
19. Paley D, Lamm BM, Purohit RM, et al. Distraction arthroplasty of the ankle–how far can you stretch the indications? [review]. Foot Ankle Clin 2008;13(3):471–84, ix.
20. Paley D, Lamm BM. Ankle joint distraction [review]. Foot Ankle Clin 2005;10(4): 685–98, ix.
21. Tarr RR, Resnick CT, Wagner KS, et al. Changes in tibiotalar joint contact areas following experimentally induced tibial angular deformities. Clin Orthop Relat Res 1985;(199):72–80.

22. Nelman K, Weiner DS, Morscher MA, et al. Multiplanar supramalleolar osteotomy in the management of complex rigid foot deformities in children. J Child Orthop 2009;3(1):39–46.

23. Staheli LT. Torsion–treatment indications [review]. Clin Orthop Relat Res 1989;(247): 61–6.

24. Lamm BM, Paley D. Deformity correction planning for hindfoot, ankle, and lower limb [review]. Clin Podiatr Med Surg 2004;21(3):305–26, v.

25. Saltzman CL, el-Khoury GY. The hindfoot alignment view. Foot Ankle Int 1995; 16(9):572–6.

26. Lamm BM, Paley D, Testani M, et al. Tarsal tunnel decompression in leg lengthening and deformity correction of the foot and ankle. J Foot Ankle Surg 2007; 46(3):201–6.

27. Mendicino RW, Catanzariti AR, Reeves CL. Percutaneous supramalleolar osteotomy for distal tibial (near articular) ankle deformities. J Am Podiatr Med Assoc 2005;95(1):72–84.

28. Coetzee JC. Surgical strategies: lateral ligament reconstruction as part of the management of varus ankle deformity with ankle replacement. Foot Ankle Int 2010;31(3):267–74.

29. Glazebrook M, Daniels T, Younger A, et al. Comparison of health-related quality of life between patients with end-stage ankle and hip arthrosis. J Bone Joint Surg Am 2008;90(3):499–505.

30. Hintermann B, Barg A, Knupp M. Corrective supramalleolar osteotomy for malunited pronation-external rotation fractures of the ankle. J Bone Joint Surg Br 2011;93(10):1367–72.

31. DeMeo PJ, Johnson EM, Chiang PP, et al. Midterm follow-up of opening-wedge high tibial osteotomy. Am J Sports Med 2010;38(10):2077–84.

32. Birmingham TB, Giffin JR, Chesworth BM, et al. Medial opening wedge high tibial osteotomy: a prospective cohort study of gait, radiographic, and patient-reported outcomes. Arthritis Rheum 2009;61(5):648–57.

33. Gomoll AH. High tibial osteotomy for the treatment of unicompartmental knee osteoarthritis: a review of the literature, indications, and technique. Phys Sportsmed 2011;39(3):45–54.

34. Waciakowski D, Urban K, Karpaš K. Valgus high tibial osteotomy - long-term results. Acta Chir Orthop Traumatol Cech 2011;78(3):225–31 [in Czech].

Osteochondral Talar Lesions and Defects

Jason L. Seiter, DPM, FACFAS[a],*, Kenneth P. Seiter Jr, DPM, AACFAS[b]

KEYWORDS

- Talar dome lesions • Ostrochondral defects • Talus fracture
- Ankle arthritis

KEY POINTS

- Talar dome lesions are known by a variety of antiquated misleading nomenclature.
- The primary leading causes of talar dome lesions are typically traumatic ankle fractures and sprains.
- Talar dome lesions may be underdiagnosed because of improper workups for ankle pain.
- Acute talar dome lesions that are minor or mild may be treated with conservative care options in some situations.
- Severe acute or chronic problematic talar dome lesions can be addressed with various surgical interventions.

INTRODUCTION

Osteochondral defects of the talar dome have been documented in the literature under various names since first being described by Alexander Monro in 1738.[1] Perhaps the name we are most familiar with, osteochondritis dissecans (OCD), coined in 1888 by Konig, is an inappropriate term nowadays given the lack of scientific support for inflammation as the causative factor in cartilage separation of talar dome lesions (TDL).[2] In addition, medical documentation of OCD is often misconstrued as the abbreviation for the mental condition of obsessive compulsive disorder, which can result in medical legal issues if misinterpreted by a third party. The term flake fracture is true in Berndt-Harty stage II, III, and IV lesions, but would be inaccurate as terminology in stage I lesions or subchondral cyst. Osteochondral lesion of the talus (OLT) is perhaps more accurate; however, it fails to address which of the 3 joints of

[a] 6224 Gordon Lane, P.O. Box 2406, Fort Smith, AR 72902, USA; [b] 11534 Kings Way Drive, P.O. Box 2406, Fort Smith, AR 72916, USA
* Corresponding author.
E-mail address: jseiter@sparks.org

Clin Podiatr Med Surg 29 (2012) 483–500
http://dx.doi.org/10.1016/j.cpm.2012.08.009
0891-8422/12/$ – see front matter © 2012 Elsevier Inc. All rights reserved.

the talus is being referred to. Regardless of antiquated or misleading nomenclature, TDL have increasingly been the focus of interest and training of many foot and ankle surgeons over the past decade.

Why the increased interest in TDL, if statistical literature indicates TDL only accounts for 0.09% of all fractures and only 1% of talus fractures?[3] The answer, simply put, is more than 1 in 20 ankle sprains and more than 1 in 4 ankle fractures will develop a TDL, which is a large volume of patients in a foot and ankle specialty practice.[2] Statistics are based on properly diagnosed cases, and fail to take into account undiagnosed incidence. Hence, the most important treatment aspect of TDL is diagnosis, so that appropriate treatment protocols can be enacted in a timely and stepwise manner. Once diagnosis is made, appropriate treatment with either conservative or surgical management can begin. By being aware of all practical treatment options and their indications, success rates, benefits, risks, and alternative options, foot and ankle specialists will be able to make an informed decision on appropriate care selection after perusing this article.

ANATOMY OF THE TALUS

It is commonly stated that the talus has poor vascularity, which is not necessarily correct. The vascularity throughout the talus is quite good, but is fragile and compromised easily with trauma, leading to poor healing potential after certain injuries. Arterial supply of the talus is via a combination of small branches from the anterior tibial artery, peroneal artery, and posterior tibial artery. The talus has no muscular coverage and therefore does not receive any indirect arterial supplementation from musculature. Given that the talus is 60% articular cartilage, the remaining surface is covered by less than 40% blood-rich periosteum. Arterial components may be compromised by traumatic events that lacerate, compress, or occlude vessels, which may occur in talar or ankle fracture or subluxation, or be disrupted in surgical incisions and fixation. Such compromise can lead to poor healing of talar bone and cartilage defects, and progress to avascular necrosis.

The talus is the key component of connection of the leg to the foot. The talus is shaped similar to the head of a dog with a long snout. The body of the talus is covered dorsally by a dome covered with cartilage, which articulates primarily with the distal tibia plafond dorsally and medially at the medial malleoli, and to a much lesser degree laterally with the fibula at the lateral malleoli to create the saddle hinge ankle joint. The inferior body of the talus articulates with the calcaneus at the subtalar joint with a combination of cartilage interfaces, the interosseus ligament, and adipose tissue of the Hoke tonsil. Distally the talar head articulates with the navicular in a modified ball-and-socket type joint. Between the talar body at the ankle and the articular head at the talonavicular joint transverses the talar neck. The talus has no muscular or tendinous attachments, but has all pedal extrinsic flexor and extrinsic extensor tendons, and both peroneal tendons passing in close proximity.

The ankle is predominately limited to motion in the sagittal plane only, but under excessive stress or compromise of ligamentous integrity the talus can also experience frontal-plane motion, which can lead to injury of the talus and ankle.

The articular surface of the talar dome is covered with a thin layer of avascular hyaline cartilage that receives nourishment from the articular fluid. Cartilage thickness ranges from 1.11 ($\pm$0.28 mm) in women and 1.35 ($\pm$0.22 mm) in men on the talar dome.[4] The hyaline cartilage consist of chondrocytes that lie in groupwise lacunae of the extracellular matrix it produces, composed of collagen, hyaluronic acid, proteoglycans, and a small amount of glycoproteins.[5]

ETIOLOGY OF OSTEOCHONDRAL TALAR LESIONS AND DEFECTS

The proposed causes of TDL have included ischemia, genetics, and infection; however, it is generally believed that trauma is the causative factor in the vast majority of lesions. If trauma is the primary cause of Talar Dome Lesions (TDL), then perhaps TDL can also stand for Traumatic Dome Lesion when appropriate. Ankle fractures have been identified as the primary cause of TDL, followed secondarily by ankle sprains. Ankle instability caused by posttraumatic causes or ligamentous laxity owing to genetic causes may lead to repetitive microtrauma due to ankle joint misalignment, and lead further to TDL development.

Berndt and Harty,[6] using cadaveric models, were able to recreate TDL and correlate lesion location with causative forces. By dorsiflexing the foot at the ankle and placing the talus in complete contact with the medial and lateral malleoli and tibial plafond followed by applying an inversion force to the foot, they were able to force the talus against its fibular articulation and create lateral TDL. In addition, by plantarflexing the foot at the ankle and placing the posterior aspect of the medial axilla of the talus in direct contact with the tibia by relaxing the collateral ligaments and placing the narrow aspect of the talar dome in the ankle joint by applying an inversion force, they were able to reproduce medial lesions. As a general rule, lateral lesions are located anteriorly and are small, shallow, and wafer-shaped because of shearing force, whereas medial lesions are located posteriorly or centrally and are larger, cup-shaped, and deep, caused by torsional impact.[7] Because of their shape, lateral lesions are more likely than medial lesions to displace.[8] Lesions may also be iatrogenically induced during surgical intervention by inappropriately inserted or manipulated arthroscopic equipment, or with internal or external fixation of ankle fractures from malpositioned drills, screws, or pins.

CLASSIFICATION OF TALAR DOME LESIONS

Classically lesions have been classified as 1 of 4 types for the past 50 years, using the Berndt and Hardy classification system based on radiographic findings.[6] In 2001, Scranton and McDermott[9] proposed their addition of a stage V lesion to the Berndt and Hardy classification system to describe a cystic lesion. Anderson and colleagues and Ferkel and colleagues[10,11] both developed classification systems using magnetic resonance imaging (MRI). Loomer and colleagues[12] developed a classification system using computed tomography (CT) imaging. Pritsch and colleagues[13] developed a classification system based on arthroscopic appearance of articular ankle cartilage.

Berndt and Harty Talar Dome Lesion Classification System

> Type I: Articular cartilage intact with underlying subchondral bone compression
> Type II: Osteochondral fragment partially detached
> Type III: Osteochondral fragment completely detached without displacement
> Type IV: Osteochondral fragment completely detached and displaced
> Type V (Scranton and McDermott): Subchondral cyst[6,9]

DIAGNOSIS OF OSTEOCHONDRAL TALAR LESIONS AND DEFECTS
History

As with all good treatment plans, it is imperative to listen to what the patient has to say subjectively. Some patients will provide too little information, whereas others will ramble on endlessly; therefore, it is important to direct the patient with appropriate questioning at times to obtain key details.

Questions Targeting Possible TDL

- Prior ankle fracture?
- Prior ankle sprain?
- Prior fall?
- Prior motor vehicle accident?
- Prior ankle surgery?
- Does the ankle hurt?
- Does the ankle swell?
- Does the ankle lock up?
- Does the ankle tend to feel unstable?
- Do multiple joints hurt, or just the ankle?
- Have you failed to improve with prior treatment?

Clinical Examination

The reason TDL are missed in some patients is perhaps because the subjective complaints of pain or ankle limitations expressed by the patient are not matched by significant objective findings recognized by the physician. Clinical examination should follow the key podiatric components of a foot and ankle examination with special care to a few details. In reviewing the vascularity, attention should be directed to identifying excessive edema, particularly when compared with the contralateral uninvolved extremity in both acute and chronic conditions. In acute conditions, bruising and formation of fracture blisters may be present, indicating additional injury such as ankle sprain or fracture. Dermatologic conditions are generally limited or nonexistent except for acute fracture blisters, or skin irritation from shoe gear or bracing owing to ankle instability. Atypical skin presentations may represent either comorbid skin issues, or differential diagnosis such as psoriatic arthritis. Neurologic findings include pain out of proportion for palpation, ambulation, and range of motion. The majority of notable issues will be related to the musculoskeletal examination. Pain with palpation of the anteromedial and anterolateral margins of the ankle joint, and possibly at the posteromedial aspect, are generally found with TDL; however, lack of pain in these areas does not exclude a TDL.[2] Range of motion actively and passively may have a clicking sound with popping sensation with or without severe pain to the patient, as the fragment or defect catches in the joint, affecting smooth normal motion. Gait analysis may demonstrate limping, guarding, and instability of the affected limb in symptomatic patients. TDL may be asymptomatic or limited in severity, with no clinical manifestations.

Imaging for Talar Dome Lesions

Plain radiography

As with most musculoskeletal injuries or complaints of pain, the initial imaging begins with standard radiographs of the involved area. Scout films should include the standard 3-view ankle and foot. Foot radiographs are used not to evaluate TDL, but rather to evaluate additional injuries or rule out other causative factors, such as fractures of the fifth metatarsal base that may be causing ankle pain. Ankle films may be shot weight bearing or non–weight bearing, depending on patient's ability to bear weight.

Additional beneficial ankle views may include a 4-cm heel lift, which plantarflexes the foot, allowing for some posterior TDL to be better visualized.[14] Stress inversion and anterior drawer may indicate ligamentous injury and can help confirm the probability of ankle sprain leading to TDL.

Radiographs, however, are limited in their ability to readily identify TDL and may not visualize 30% to 43% of lesions.[3,14,15] Plain radiographs are limited by their ability to predominately only visualize osseous bone structures and are not able to visual non-calcified cartilage structures. As a result, TDL that only involve cartilage surfaces may not readily be identified until they progress with time to cause cystic bone lesions to appear as radiopaque lesions. Serial radiographs may be needed with several weeks to months between series before a TDL is evident.

Computed tomography

CT examinations have been considered by many to be the preferred method of definitely evaluating TDL before surgical intervention, as the lesion can be evaluated in multiple planes. CT allows for detailed evaluation of the osseous component of the TDL to measure lesion size and location. To obtain optimal imaging of a TDL with CT, the imaging protocol calls for ultrahigh-resolution axial slices with 0.3-mm increments and 0.6-mm thickness, with 1-mm coronal and sagittal multiplanar reconstruction.[8] CT is limited due to its decreased ability to characterize and visualize the cartilage component of the TDL, which can be rather problematic when evaluating Berndt-Harty stage I lesions.[16] CT can generally be performed on a larger population of patients than can MRI, because one is able to perform CT on patients who have pacemaker/defibrillator implantation or ferrous or unknown metal foreign bodies, both of which are contra-indications for MRI. CT may be the preferred advanced diagnostic imaging method if additional osseous structures such as the tibia and fibula are in question, such as in a comminuted ankle fracture. CT scans are generally preferred when a TDL is already known to be present and surgical intervention is pending.

Magnetic resonance imaging

MRI is considered the preferred tool for diagnosis and preoperative planning for TDL by the majority of remaining physicians. Like CT, MRI allows the lesion to be evaluated in multiple planes. MRI has the ability not only to visualize osseous defects (perhaps not to the degree of CT) but also to give greater detail with regard to cartilage integrity. Unlike CT, MRI generally allows Berndt-Harty stage I lesions to be detected, and findings have been found to correlate closely with arthroscopically visualized findings for cartilage defects.[16] MRI may be the preferred advanced diagnostic imaging method if additional soft-tissue structures such as the ankle ligaments are in question, such as in a severe sprain. MRI scans are generally preferred when a TDL is suspected but not already definitely identified.

Bone scintigraphy (3-phase bone scan)

Bone scintigraphy can be used as a screening tool to help detect the potential presence of TDL when plain radiography is inconclusive. Studies have shown bone scintigraphy to be 94% sensitive and 96% specific for TDL when abnormal uptake in the talar dome was noted on at least one view by Urman and colleagues.[17] Although bone scintigraphy may be helpful in indicating whether a TDL is present, it provides little information on size, location, and severity, and therefore should be followed by a more definitive imaging modality such as CT or MRI before surgical planning.

Arthroscopy

Ankle arthroscopy has become perhaps the definitive way to evaluate, and many times treat TDL. Arthroscopy allows not only direct visualization of the TDL but also allows for manipulation of the lesion to provide further diagnostic quality for the lesion. Many, but not all TDL can be treated with arthroscopic techniques such as debridement, microfracture, and subchondral drilling at the same time as arthroscopic visualization. Arthroscopy may be performed at the time of initial surgical intervention, such as during open reduction and internal fixation of an ankle fracture, or may be performed after other advanced imaging techniques including CT or MRI, so that the lesion size and location has been predetermined. Arthroscopic evaluation can be limited by the location or depth of the lesion or by the surgical expertise of the individual performing the arthroscopic examination.

CONSERVATIVE NONOPERATIVE TREATMENT OF OSTEOCHONDRAL TALAR LESIONS AND DEFECTS

Conservative nonoperative care should generally be the initial line of care for most TDL. Surgery is necessitated when a patient has failed the standard length and course of nonoperative care. Berndt-Harty stage I and II TDL have the best prognosis, with 90% resolution with nonoperative care, and can be managed nonsurgically for up to 12 months before initiating surgical options.[16,18] Expert recommendations from long-term follow-up studies by individuals treating all 4 Berndt-Harty grade lesions indicate that stage I or II medial or lateral, and stage III medial lesions can initially be treated with conservative nonoperative care; however, stage III lateral and stage IV medial or lateral lesions should proceed to surgical intervention.[7,18]

Protective Weight-Bearing Devices and Strapping

Bracing, strapping, or taping combined with protected early ankle motion may allow for Berndt-Harty stage I TDL to resolve to tolerable levels after several weeks to months. Berndt-Harty stage II lesions may resolve with 1 to 1 and a half months of immobilization with a 3D immobilization boot, CAM walker boot, or short leg walking cast; the same treatment for up to 4 and a half months has also been shown to be beneficial in stage III medial lesions.[7]

Oral Nonsteroidal Anti-Inflammatories and Oral Steroids

Nonsteroidal anti-inflammatory drugs (NSAIDs) may provide significant pain and swelling reduction by reducing associated synovitis and capsulitis of the ankle joint. As with all NSAID use, care needs to be considered in certain groups because of cardiac and renal risk, and potential gastrointestinal (GI) ulceration and bleeding with long-term use. Alternatively a course of oral steroids may be initiated in the short term to reduce any significant synovitis and capsulitis either before NSAIDs, or if initial NSAIDs fail to provide relief. Oral steroids should be avoided or used with caution in diabetic patients or if surgical intervention is planned, owing to their potential to elevate blood sugar, delay wound healing, and increase the risk of postoperative infection.

Ankle Steroid Injections

Steroid injections into the ankle joint can be both therapeutic and diagnostic with their ability to rapidly reduce pain and swelling. The exact amount and type of steroid with or without additional compounds such as local anesthetic is generally based on a physician's own clinical experience. Local steroid injections are generally tolerated much better than oral steroids by diabetics in regard of glucose elevation, and are generally safer than oral NSAIDs in patients with cardiac, renal, or GI issues. Steroid injections do have some concern because of the potential delay in wound healing and the increased risk of postoperative infection; however, the joint is generally well flushed out of remaining steroid with procedures such as arthroscopy, making it a moot concern. Failure of the TDL lesion to improve, even short term, may indicate that the TDL is either deep or cystic, or that additional or alternative abnormality may be present. The patient should be cautioned to avoid excessive activity that may result in further injury, as the body's ability to perceive pain with further injury may be remarkably suppressed.

Hyaluronate Ankle Injections

Injections of hyaluronic acid into the joint have been used by orthopedists, with good reported results, over the past few decades for the treatment of arthritis, predominately of the knee, but now with potential clinical indications for other large joints. Numerous well-respected published reports can be readily found indicating the effectiveness of hyaluronic acid on variable anatomic joints other than the knee; however, the manufacturer, Food and Drug Administration, and most insurance providers indicate its use only in the knee. Hyaluronic acid was first discovered by Meyer and Palmer in 1934, and since that time has been progressively studied in both composition and use in humans. Hyaluronic acid is naturally produced in joints by chondrocytes in cartilage and synoviocytes to provide viscoelasticity to joint fluid and critical components to the extracellular matrix of articular cartilage.[19] Injecting hyaluronic acid into joints with osteoarthritis has been shown to augment the flow of synovial fluid, inhibit the degradation and normalize the synthesis of endogenous hyaluronic acid, in addition to relieving joint pain.[19,20] The ankle injections have been recommended to be performed once a week for a 3- or 5-week course.[19,21] Studies have predominately focused around the use of hyaluronan injections alone as conservative nonoperative care, but new research has been released stating the benefits of injections postsurgically after microfracture of TDL, indicating better outcomes than with microfracture of TDL alone.[21,22] Injected hyaluronic acid is absent within days of injection; however, the clinical benefit tends to last 6 or more months.[19,21] The long-term benefits can vary among manufacturers, and range from 60 days to 22 weeks. Off-label use of hyaluronic acid in the ankle joint may provide reduction in TDL symptoms if the patient and physician are willing to accept the associated out-of-pocket cost and potential off-label legal risk.

Physical Therapy

Physical therapy (PT) may provide adjunctive therapy to TDL by aiding patients in better gait with assistive devices for extended periods of time, strapping of the ankle, increased ankle range of motion, and reduction in pain and swelling of the ankle. In addition, PT may be able to increase ankle stability in conditions such as ankle sprain and lateral ankle instability, which may be contributing factors to ankle pain.

Pulsed Electromagnetic Field Treatment

Pulsed electromagnetic fields (PEMF) have been used over the past 2 decades for the treatment of bone fractures, predominately in nonunions or patients at risk for nonunions. PEMF use for osteoarthritis has been limited, and such studies have been predominately limited to the spine and knee, which did show significant reduction in pain, increased function, and reduced morning stiffness.[23,24] A study by Bloom and colleagues[23] reported a 73.3% success rate among 60 patients treated for microtrabecular fracture of the talus with or without a Berndt-Harty stage I or II TDL using PEMF for 3 months after having failed at least 3 months of protected weight bearing, casting, or CAM walker. Further published studies would need to be undertaken to definitively confirm or refute the benefit of PEMF for TDL as a nonsurgical modality in its own right. PEMF historically has been used and indicated for the incorporation of bone grafts after fracture repair, and from this reasoning may provide better and faster healing after fresh frozen allograft osteochondral block implants into the talus.

SURGICAL TREATMENT OF OSTEOCHONDRAL TALAR LESIONS AND DEFECTS
Arthroscopic Procedures

Arthroscopy can be used to treat the majority of TDL with debridement, microfracturing, and drilling through cannulated instrumentation and visualization, and has become the gold standard for treatment of most TDL, or at least the first line of stepwise surgical intervention. Typically either a 4.0-mm or 2.7-mm videoarthroscope is used for visualization, and an assortment of microfracture picks, curettes, burs, probes, osteotomes, drills, and punches of the surgeon's preference are used to resect and repair the TDL. Inflow and outflow of fluid may be accomplished by either pump and suction or gravity alone as per surgeon preference. A thigh tourniquet or epinephrine injected into the ankle joint may be used to decrease an obstructed field of view from active bleeding.

Multiple portal exposures, anterior and posterior, have been described including anterior medial, anterior central, anterior lateral, posterior medial, posterior central (transachilles tendon), and posterior lateral. Despite the multiple portal techniques listed the in literature, the anterior medial and anterior lateral portals are the standard because of their ability to provide exposure to medial, lateral, and central lesions, and reduce the risk of injury to major neurovascular and tendenous structures. If choosing alternative higher-risk portals, the benefits should outweigh the risk and should be reserved for surgeons with advanced arthroscopic experience.

Some investigators recommend a medial malleolar osteotomy when dealing with medial TDL owing to their central posterior sites, whereas various surgical techniques aimed at approaching medial TDL in an effort to avoid osteotomy have been described throughout the literature. Many posteromedial TDL do not have to be treated by malleolar osteotomy but can be treated arthroscopically by bringing the foot into hyperplantar flexion.[25–28] In addition, noninvasive ankle straps can be used to distend the ankle joint with straps and post secured to the operating table to maintain increased joint space throughout the procedure. Further ankle distraction can be accomplished by relaxing the posterior muscle group by elevating the thigh with a thigh holder, affixed to a rod, to the operating table, and partially flexing both the hip and knee.

Arthroscopic lavage and debridement removes the catabolic cytokines and loose bodies from the ankle, reducing the cause of mechanical symptoms. Small, chronic, symptomatic lesions often benefit from lavage and debridement, which make no attempt to repair or replace damaged articular cartilage. Chondroplasty, normally used in the knee, may be used to remove a cartilage flap to a stable base. Lavage alone has yielded variable short-term results. In a review of the literature, excisional debridement alone of TDL had the lowest success rate (38%) of any surgical procedure, ranging from 30% to 100% among studies. Excision and curettage had a success rate of 76% with a range of 53% to 100% among studies.[29] The success rate for arthroscopic procedures (84%) was higher than for open procedures (63%).

The rationale of microfracturing and drilling is to partially destroy the calcified zone that is most often present and create multiple openings within the subchondral bone. Intraosseous blood vessels are disrupted, and the release of growth factors leads to the formation of a fibrin clot and yields a fibrocartilaginous matrix composed of chondroblasts, chondrocytes, fibrocytes, and an unorganized matrix that protects the surface from excessive loading.[30–32] There are currently no pharmacologic methods for inducing expression of type II (hyaline) cartilage; therefore, these methods result in a fibrocartilage covering that is biomechanically inferior to the native hyaline cartilage. However, the literature shows this technique to provide good pain relief in short-term and medium-term follow-up studies. Microfracture and drilling cause bleeding as a result of violating of the subchondral bone. Thermal necrosis is a potential complication of drilling. Across 21 studies using excision, curettage, and drilling, an overall 86% rate of successful outcomes has been reported.[29] Partial weight bearing and early range-of-motion exercises and are generally recommended and are considered to be essential for rapid recovery.

Results of excision alone are improved with the addition of curettage and furthermore with drilling, as discerned on review of the literature. In addition, arthroscopic results appear to be superior to open procedures. Early results of microfracture of the talus have demonstrated high (93%), excellent, or good results.[33–37]

Arthroscopic debridement techniques are generally not recommended in large cartilage defects (greater than 1.5 cm^2) and lesions with large or deep cysts of 7 mm or greater.[38,39]

Arthrotomy

Open arthrotomy may be used when direct exposure of the talar dome is deemed necessary to allow for increased visibility that cannot be obtained through an arthroscope and that does not warrant medial or lateral malleolar osteotomy exposure. Open direct exposure allows for larger instrumentation and the ability to apply grafts that are not amenable to arthroscopic technique. Incision placement is generally in the same location as for arthroscope portals (anterior medial and anterior lateral), taking care not to injure the underlying neurovascular and tendinous structures. Occasionally an arthroscopic procedure will develop complications from failed equipment or poor visualization, and needs to be converted to open arthrotomy, which can be accomplished by extending the portals into vertical extended incisions. Alternatively, a single anterior central incision can be made by incising a longer vertical incision and retracting medially and laterally, similar to the exposure for total ankle replacement.

Some surgeons may use variations of open arthrotomy to incorporate additional surgical interventions and procedures using alternative incision patterns, most notably to evaluate for TDL when performing initial open reduction and internal fixation of an acute ankle fracture. An arthroscope camera or tools may also be used through open incision for evaluation and debridement without the standard inflow and outflow of wet arthroscopy.

Malleolar Osteotomy

Medial or lateral malleolar osteotomies may be used when the TDL is too far posterior for arthroscopic debridement and repair or when a large osteochondral graft or artificial graft is being implanted. Osteochondral autograft and allograft plugs need to be implanted perpendicular to the talar dome joint surface, which can generally only be obtained geometrically by an osteotomy, unless anterior enough to allow for arthrotomy. All fresh frozen talus allograft en bloc procedures require malleolar osteotomy to allow exposure for resection of the compromised recipient talus, and implantation and fixation of this type of large graft.

Medial malleolar osteotomies are created at the intersection between the medial malleolus and tibial plafond, whereas lateral malleolar osteotomies are created in a similar fashion just below the syndesmosis, taking care not to disrupt it. Often the drill holes for the malleolar osteotomy fixation are predrilled before creation of the osteotomy to allow for ease of fixation when closing the osteotomy. Osteotomies are typically either oblique or incorporate a stabilizing shelf using a chevron or "Z" cut to increase stability and reduce risk of nonunion or malunion. Alternatively, in acute fractures the fracture line itself may allow for direct visualization or insertion of an arthroscope to evaluate the talar dome at a given time before standard open reduction and internal fixation of the ankle fracture.

Retrograde Talar Drilling

In 2001, Scranton and McDermott proposed their addition of a stage V lesion to the Berndt-Hardy classification system to describe a cystic lesion that was not originally included in the prior 4-stage classification system.[9] Cystic lesion etiology remains unclear; however, one theory postulates that synovial fluid under pressure erodes subchondral bone after development of a fissure in the cartilage. It remains unknown at what point in the development of a TDL a cyst occurs. Cystic lesions with an intact overlying hyaline cartilage cape create a unique challenge in attempting to preserve the original cartilage while repairing the underlying cyst, which generally is not amenable to intra-articular procedures.

Retrograde drilling addresses the issue of a cyst by approaching the cyst through the body of the talus itself while keeping the overlying cartilage intact. The drill may enter either through the wall of the body of the talus or through the sinus tarsi. Appropriate drill placement may be performed with noninvasive aiming guides that point from the lesion to the outer skin, or more simply by passing a minimally invasive guide wire through the articular cartilage of the TDL and cyst through the talar body to the outer portion of the foot for drill placement. Wire and drill placement may be confirmed with intraoperative fluoroscopy. The cyst is drilled through then back-filled with a bone void filler of the surgeon's preference, typically demineralized bone matrix putty, via syringe.

Osteochondral Autograft Transplant System and Mosaicplasty

The most successful technique in treating large, full-thickness loss of articular cartilage with or without cysts and failed TDL remains controversial. Restorative techniques have been shown to be capable of restoring the articular hyaline cartilage surface, including defects larger than 2 cm.[38,39]

Osteochondral autografting includes the osteochondral autograft transfer system (OATS) of single graft plugs and mosaicplasty of multiple smaller graft plugs. The theoretical advantage of these techniques is restoration of a normal hyaline cartilage surface using the patient's own cells. These techniques use a plug of cartilage and associated subchondral bone that is harvested either locally or from a distal site such as the lesser weight-bearing femoral condyle of the ipsilateral knee, and implanted into the prepared osteochondral defect on the talar dome. When the knee is precluded as a donor site, use of small autologous grafts from the anterior talus can be considered. Mosaicplasty is preferred because it provides a better congruency to the talar dome contour and surface area defect, with less donor-site morbidity. Fibrocartilage is reported to develop in the residual defect spaces between the multiple round plug interfaces, resulting in a mottled patch work of both hyaline and fibrocartilage when performing mosaicplasty. By contrast, single plug grafts develop predominately or solely hyaline cartilage, although donor-site morbidity may be greater because of harvest of a single larger plug.

In 2003, 63 consecutive patients with TDL treated with mosaicplasty were reviewed at an average follow-up of 5.8 years.[40] The mean patient age was 25.2 years and the average defect was 1 cm in diameter. The average number of grafts used was 3 (range, 1–7 grafts). The primary donor site was the superior medial edge of the medial femoral condyle. The location and presumed etiology of the lesions was not provided. At final follow-up, using the Hannover scoring system, the author reported 47 excellent, 11 good, 3 moderate, and 2 poor results. Biopsy at second-look arthroscopy revealed type II collagen and proteoglycans consistent with articular cartilage. The investigators concluded that early-term and medium-term results of mosaicplasty were encouraging.

Autologous Chondrocyte Implantation

Autologous chondrocyte implantation (ACI) is a 2-procedure technique, originally recommended for the knee, which necessitates a graft-harvesting procedure to obtain 200 to 300 mg of autologous chondrocytes from the superior medial or lateral femoral condyle or the intercondylar ridge of the knee.[41,42] The in vitro cultured autologous chondrocytes are isolated and proliferated for at least 4 weeks before reimplantation through an arthrotomy. ACI is typically reserved for lesions larger than 10 mm in diameter, well-contained stage III and IV defects, large lesions with extensive subchondral cystic changes, lesions refractory to treatment with other reparative techniques, and failed previous surgery. Ideally the patient is between 15 and 55 years old and has no malalignment, degenerative joint disease, or instability of the joint. The procedure is contraindicated in bipolar (kissing) lesions involving both the tibia and talus. Because the technique requires procurement of cells from a donor site, there is an associated risk of donor-site morbidity.[41,42]

Subsequent to the lesion undergoing debridement, an autologous periosteal flap is harvested and secured with 5-0 or 6-0 Vicryl over the implanted cultured chondrocytes and sealed with fibrin glue. Implantation of the cells and sewing of the periosteal flap is not amenable to arthroscopic surgery. In cases of associated bone loss with cystic changes, the bone defect is bone-grafted and covered with a periosteal patch with its cambium side facing the cartilage. To create a space for the cells, a second periosteal patch is sewn over the first patch, with its cambium side facing the bone. ACI creates hyaline-like cartilage in the defect and can be used in conjunction with bone grafting to fill larger defects.[41,42]

Fresh Frozen Talus Allograft En Bloc

Fresh frozen talus allograft en bloc is a practical option for a subset of TDL with location of lesions on the curvature of the talus shoulder, size greater than 10 mm, or failed prior surgical intervention with osteochondral drilling and microfracture or osteochondral plugs. The patient's anatomy and measurements of the talus and defect are predetermined by advanced diagnostic imaging, with CT being the preferred modality. A request is made to the tissue bank for a fresh frozen talus allograft en bloc of certain size and characteristics that best match the patient's needs. A periodic wait may or may not occur depending on the given request. Notification is made to the surgeon as to when a graft will be available, to allow for scheduling and workup of the patient within 48 to 72 hours of finding a suitable donor to allow for graft harvest and preparation by the tissue bank. A medial or lateral osteotomy is performed to gain appropriate patient talus exposure and resection of the problematic area. The corresponding donor talus is cut to exact specifications to allow for near identical fit of the en bloc allograft composed of both viable articular cartilage and corticocancellous bone. Fixation is with either absorbable fixation or countersunk metal screws. The joint is irrigated, soft-tissue structures repaired, and osteotomy fixated. Range-of-motion exercises begin at the surgeon's discretion, generally after the soft-tissue envelope heals within 2 to 3 weeks. Weight bearing is typically non–weight bearing in cast, removable cast boot, or splint for 4 to 8 weeks to allow both the allograft bone to incorporate into the recipient talus and the malleolar osteotomy to heal and stabilize. Protected weight bearing transitions to return to regular shoe gear limited to low impact, until cleared by the surgeon to progress to athletic activity several months postoperatively if there are no complications.

Benefits of frozen talus allograft en bloc are most notably the lack of donor-site morbidity and the ability to use anatomy and geometry that most closely match the patient's own talus. In general, fresh frozen talus allograft en bloc is the last procedure option in attempting to avoid ankle fusion or total ankle arthroplasty and their associated limitations.

The risks of this procedure include reabsorption and failure of the graft to incorporate, which results in subchondral collapse and fragmentation of the graft.[43] Osteochondral allografts may develop no viable cartilage because of decreased viability of cells at the time of transfer. Decreased chondrocyte viability occurs with each hour of time. Typically the talus is harvested within 24 hours of the donor's death while performing a background donor health disease assessment, processed and frozen, then implanted into the recipient within 3 days after harvest. The possibility of disease transfer, though low, does exist. Malleolar osteotomy nonunion, malunion, and shortening are associated risks of obtaining surgical exposure of the talus. Decreased ankle range of motion with pain can occur if the fresh frozen talus allograft en bloc is too large for the ankle mortis during dorsiflexion.

Fresh Frozen Talus Allograft Using OATS

Fresh frozen talus allograft using OATS for TDL is a concept of performing osteochondral plug transfer similar to that performed with the previously described autograft OATS procedures without the donor-site morbidity. Rather than harvesting plugs from the patient's own knee, a fresh frozen talus allograft is used as the donor site. Principles of allograft OATS are followed in identical fashion to autograft OATS regarding the patient's talar dome exposure with malleolar osteotomies and talus preparation including removal of TDL with the OATS system or burr. The donor graft is also harvested by the OATS; however, rather than harvesting from the lateral femoral condyle the graft is harvested from the same geographic area on the allograft talus to match the anatomy of the recipient TDL drilled defect. The allograft plug can be rather large, as there is no concern about donor-site morbidity; however, mosaicplasty may be performed if the lesion is larger than the OATS harvester. The fresh frozen talus allograft is obtained from the tissue bank in the same manner as for fresh frozen talus allograft en bloc, with the same associated delays and preoperative planning.

Benefits of the fresh frozen talus allograft OATS procedure are most notably the lack of donor-site morbidity and the ability to use anatomy and geometry that most closely match the patient's own talus.

The risks of this procedure are similar to those described for both fresh frozen talus allograft en bloc and autograft OATS, with the exception of donor-site morbidity to the knee.

Postoperative protocol is similar to that of autograft OATS procedures with regard to weight bearing, range of motion, and progression activity at the discretion of the surgeon.

Juvenile Allograft Cartilage

Arthroscopic debridement, subchondral drilling, and microfracture remains the mainstay of TDL surgical intervention; however, this intervention is limited by the fact that it results in the development of fibrocartilage rather than the desired hyaline cartilage at the intervention site. Until recently, only autografts with their associated donor-site morbidity or the use of large open techniques to implant allograft wedges or plugs had the ability to produce the desired hyaline cartilage at the location of intervention.

DeNovo NT (Zimmer, Warsaw, IN) is now being used by some surgeons in the ankle, in addition to other locations including the hallux, knee, hip, shoulder, and elbow, to regenerate hyaline-like cartilage.[44] DeNovo NT consists of particulated human juvenile cartilage with living cells recovered from juvenile donor joints. After implantation to the articular defect the graft is secured with a fibrin adhesive, negating the need for harvesting a periosteal flap.[44]

Alan Ng, at the American College of Foot and Ankle Surgeons 2012 Annual Scientific Conference in San Antonio, Texas, presented a technique he also published with Kruse, Paden, and Stone in 2012 on the use of DeNovo NT juvenile allograft cartilage implanted atop a TDL using an arthroscopic technique to implant and grow hyaline-like cartilage.[45,46] After using a standard wet arthroscopic technique to debride, subchondrally drill, and microfracture the TDL, the joint is drained and dried of fluid so as not to wash or irrigate away the flakes of juvenile allograft cartilage. Using the arthroscope instrument portal, the tiny flakes of DeNovo NT juvenile allograft cartilage are placed onto the prepared defect, smoothed into an appropriate layer, then sealed into place with fibrin glue. Postoperative care comprised non–weight bearing in a bivalve for 4 weeks, then a removable cast boot with non–weight bearing and range-of-motion exercise for 2 weeks. At 6 weeks, weight bearing in a cast boot for 2 weeks was initiated, until return of regular shoe gear over the following 2 weeks. Activity level progressed over a 6-month course to eventually include strenuous activities such as jogging with no reported pain. At 2 years postoperatively the patient reported no pain and full range of motion of the involved ankle. This technique is new and unique for the treatment of TDL, with only one known published report of a single case with reported excellent outcome; further published studies with larger patient populations will ultimately be required to determine the overall effectiveness of this new procedure for widespread use among other surgeons.

Unipolar Metallic Partial Implants

Unipolar metallic partial talar dome implants are a new and upcoming option for failed primary treatment of TDL. In 2007, Arthrosurface (Franklin, MA) developed HemiCAP, a set of 15 rigid metallic contoured 2-piece stemmed implants with offset sizes, in an attempt to provide surgeons with a means of replacing the medial talar dome with an implant that matches the geometry.[47] Benefits of the procedure were to provide a means of replacing the defect without any secondary morbidity sites associated with autografts, risk of disease transmission with allografts, or time delay for incorporation of biological grafts. Access for the HemiCAP implant is through the use of an osteotomy at the intersection between the medial malleolus and tibial plafond, as this allows for the appropriate and critical positioning of the guide wire, articular measurements to determine implant shape, screw post placement, implant trials, and final articular implant placement.[47] Concerns exist about the possibility of the hard metallic implant plowing into the softer articular surface of the tibia if too proud, or collapse of the adjacent articular cartilage if too recessed.[47–50] A study by van Bergen and colleagues[47] used cadaveric lower limbs to determine the contact pressure of the opposite tibial cartilage, and found them to be acceptable when the implant was recessed to a mean level of 0.45 mm (standard deviation 0.18 mm). In addition, the same investigators reported that during the study they were able to find an appropriate anatomic fit and contour among the 15 implant sizes available from HemiCAP. Concerns have been expressed both about this published work and, recently, verbally at an expert panel discussion at the American College of Foot and Ankle Surgeons 2012 Scientific Conference about the need for clinical trials with patients reporting good long-term outcomes before this procedure can be recommended as a viable treatment option.[45,47]

Ankle Arthrodiastasis

Ankle arthrodiastasis, also referred to as ankle distraction arthroplasty, may offer improvement in TDL as either primary or ancillary surgical treatment. The patient receives application of a hinged Ilizarov-style ringed external fixator that linearly distracts the ankle joint while allowing ankle range of motion. The frame is created by transfixing a ring or plate proximal to the ankle in the tibia with half pins and transfixing a second ring or plate distal to the ankle with smooth or olive wires through the talus and calcaneus. The 2 plates are separated by threaded rods that allow for distraction to desired surgeon parameters, generally 5 mm to 7 mm, which reduces contact pressures between articular cartilage of the talus and tibia. Hinges are anatomically aligned to allow range-of-motion exercise or weight bearing. Weight bearing generally begins on the day of surgery, whereas range-of-motion exercise is typically delayed until 2 weeks postoperatively. The frame and distraction it provides are kept in place for approximately 12 weeks, at which time they may be removed and the patient treated with walking boot and PT until the desired pain reduction and gait allows regular shoe gear and increased activity.

The theory behind ankle arthrodiastasis is to allow for intermittent cyclical flow of synovial fluid joint pressures, to allow cartilage and osseous healing while limiting or eliminating mechanical stress and shear forces from axial loading that impedes healing of cartilage and bone cyst.[51]

Adjunctive surgical intervention may include arthroscopic debridement, microfracture, and subchondral drilling, or autograft or allograft procedures. Adjunctive nonsurgical treatments may include intra-articular steroid or hyaluronic acid injections and PT.

The most notable risk of ankle arthrodiastasis with external fixation is pin-tract cellulitis infection at the wires in the foot or half pins in the tibia, which, if treated early with antibiotics, generally resolve readily. Even with appropriate pin care, pin-tract infection is possible given the 12-week duration of the external fixator. If untreated, pin-tract infections can lead to osteomyelitis of the tibia or abscess of the foot. Less common but still of concern is fracture of the tibia from half pins. Fracture of the tibia may occur during weight bearing if the frame is not properly aligned, or result from a postoperative fall caused by compromised gait.

Total Ankle Replacement and Ankle Fusion

Total ankle replacement (TAR) and ankle fusion are neither the primary nor secondary choice of treatment for TDL, and are reserved as the definitive final treatment option when all else has failed. Indications for TAR and ankle fusion include advanced bipolar arthritis of both the talus and tibia articular surfaces, multiple failed attempts at stepwise TDL intervention including OATS or en bloc talus allografts, patient's refusal of allograft procedures for religious or spiritual reasons, or chronic pain despite previous surgical intervention.

TAR had a previous poor history in prior decades in the United States, and is now more aggressively regulated by federal regulations regarding which type of implants and which manufacturers' products are approved in the United States market. As a result of better regulation, physician education, and research; today's total ankle implants provide a safe and reliable option to preserve ankle motion and function by sacrificing the joint with a joint-destructive replacement procedure. Like most artificial joint implants, implant life is limited to 1 or 2 decades before the implant begins to fail and requires replacement, which is problematic in the young patient who might require several revisional implants in a lifetime. Because TDL tend to occur in younger active individuals and TAR is generally intended for seniors with limited-impact activities, TAR is generally reserved for when all else fails for TDL in older, less active, nonobese patients.

Ankle fusion is generally considered by most foot and ankle surgeons to be the gold-standard definitive procedure for uncontrollable pain from advanced ankle arthritis after alternative joint-sparing surgical interventions have failed. TDL generally do not result in ankle fusion unless the lesion is excessively large or encompasses both the talus and tibia, there are uncorrectable ankle instability issues, or prior intervention has resulted in a septic joint. Because ankle fusion is a joint-destructive procedure and does not preserve any ankle function other than stability, it is a poor choice for TDL intervention, except as a last resort to provide pain relief after all else has failed.

SUMMARY

TDL are becoming more prevalent in foot and ankle practices, perhaps not because of increased frequency in a historical perspective as regards occurrence, but rather because of better diagnosis through clinical correlation and confirmation with diagnostic imaging performed by today's foot and ankle specialist. Clinical suspicion arising from increased knowledge will lead to appropriate workup with appropriate imaging to confirm TDL location, size, and severity. Armed with this information the physician can begin conservative care or, when appropriate, proceed directly to surgical intervention. Arthroscopy has been clearly indicated to be the primary and perhaps the most important surgical skill that needs to be mastered by the foot and ankle surgeon treating TDL, as it is generally the first line of treatment and typically the definitive way of addressing the lesion in the majority of cases to confirm the lesion, perform debridement, and at times augment the lesion with appropriate biological materials. In addition, alternative exposure techniques to the talar dome using arthrotomy, osteotomy, and retrograde drilling must be mastered to allow for access to recessed lesions, wide resections, and larger allografts and implants. Noninvasive and invasive ancillary and augmented techniques may substantially improve the outcome of the primary procedure when appropriate, particularly in revisional procedures. Surgeons have the responsibility of performing procedures that are evidence based to achieve a good outcome, but researchers have the responsibility of pushing the envelope to develop the tools, medications, and techniques needed to allow these good outcomes to be possible.

ACKNOWLEDGMENTS

Special thanks are extended to Grace Anderson of AHEC, Sparks Regional Medical Center medical library for her help in the literature search and in obtaining medical journal papers for review to make this article possible.

REFERENCES

1. Monroe A. Part of the cartilage of the joint, separated and ossified. In: Medical essays and observations, vol. IV. Edinburgh (United Kingdom): Ruddimans; 1738. p. 19.
2. Grossman J, Lyons M. A review of osteochondral lesions of the talus. Clin Podiatr Med Surg 2009;26:205–26.
3. Flick AB, Gould N. Osteochondritis dissecans of the talus (transchondral fractures of the talus): review of the literature and new surgical approach for medial dome lesions. Foot Ankle 1985;5(4):165–85.

4. Sugimoto K, Takakura Y, Kumai T, et al. Cartilage thickness of the talar dome. Arthroscopy 2005;21:401–4.
5. Van Dijk C, Reilingh M, Zengerink M, et al. Osteochondral defects in the ankle: why painful? Knee Surg Sports Traumatol Arthrosc 2010;18:570–80.
6. Berndt AL, Harty M. Transchondral fractures (osteochondral dissecans) of the talus. J Bone Joint Surg Am 1959;41:988–1020.
7. Canale ST, Belding RH. Osteochondral lesions of the talus. J Bone Joint Surg Am 1980;62(1):97–102.
8. van Bergen C, de Leeuw P, van Dijk C. Treatment of osteochondral lesions of the talus. Rev Chir Orthop Reparatrice Appar Mot 2008;945:S398–408.
9. Scranton PE Jr, McDermott JE. Treatment of type V osteochondral lesions of the talus with ipsilateral knee osteochondral autografts. Foot Ankle Int 2001;22(5):380–4.
10. Anderson IF, Crichton KJ, Grattan-Smith T, et al. Osteochondral fractures of the dome of the talus. J Bone Joint Surg Am 1989;71:1143–52.
11. Ferkel RD, Flannigan BD, Elkins BS. Magnetic resonance imaging of the foot and ankle: correlation of normal anatomy with pathologic conditions. Foot Ankle 1991; 11:289–305.
12. Loomer R, Fischer C, Lloyd-Smith R, et al. Osteochondral lesions of the talus. Am J Sports Med 1993;21(1):13–9.
13. Pritsch M, Horoshovski H, Farine I. Arthroscopic treatment of osteochondral lesions of the talus. J Bone Joint Surg Am 1986;68:862–5.
14. Verhagen RA, Maas M, Dijkgraaf MG. Prospective study on diagnostic strategies in osteochondral lesions of the talus. Is MRI superior to helical CT? J Bone Joint Surg Br 2005;87(1):41–6.
15. Hepple S, Winson IG, Glew D. Osteochondral lesions of the talus: a revised classification. Foot Ankle Int 1999;20(12):789–93.
16. Schachter AK, Chen AL, Reddy PD, et al. Osteochondral lesions of the talus. J Am Acad Orthop Surg 2005;13:152–8.
17. Urman M, Ammann W, Sisler J, et al. The role of bone scintigraphy in the evaluation of talar dome fractures. J Nucl Med 1991;32:2241–4.
18. Pettine KA, Morrey BF. Osteochondral fractures of the talus—a long-term follow-up. J Bone Joint Surg 1987;69B:89–92.
19. Mei-Dan O, Kish B, Shabat S, et al. Treatment of osteoarthritis of the ankle by intra-articular injections of hyaluronic acid. J Am Podiatr Med Assoc 2010; 100(2):93–100.
20. Rydell N, Balazs EA. Effect of intra-articular injection of hyaluronic acid on the clinical symptoms of osteoarthritis and on granulation tissue formation. Clin Orthop Relat Res 1971;80:25.
21. Sun S, Hsu C, Sun H, et al. The effect of three weekly intra-articular injections of hyaluronate on pain, function, and balance in patients with unilateral ankle arthritis. J Bone Joint Surg Am 2011;93:1720–6.
22. Doral M, Bilge O, Donmez G, et al. Treatment of osteochondral lesions of the talus with microfracture technique and postoperative hyaluronan injection. Knee Surg Sports Traumatol Arthrosc 2011;20(7):1398–403.
23. Bloom T, Renard R, Yalamanchili P, et al. Stimulation of ankle cartilage: other emerging technologies (cellular, electromagnetic, etc.). Foot Ankle Clin 2008;13(3):363–79.
24. Zizic TM, Hoffman KC, Holt PA, et al. The treatment of osteoarthritis of the knee with pulsed electrical stimulation. J Rheumatol 1995;22:1757–61.
25. Assenmacher JA, Kelikian AS, Gottlob C, et al. Arthroscopically assisted autologous osteochondral transplantation for osteochondral lesions of the talar dome: an MRI and clinical follow-up study. Foot Ankle Int 2001;22(7):544–51.

26. Hangody L, Kish G, Karpati Z, et al. Treatment of osteochondritis dissecans of the talus: use of the mosaicplasty technique- preliminary report. Foot Ankle Int 1997; 18(10):628–34.
27. Hangody L, Kish G, Modis L, et al. Mosaicplasty for the treatment of osteochondritis dissecans of the talus-two to seven year results in 36 patients. Foot Ankle Int 2001;22(7):552–8.
28. Petersen L, Brittberg M, Lindahl A. Autologous chondrocyte transplantation of the ankle. Foot Ankle Clin 2003;8(2):291–303.
29. Verhagen RA, Struijs PA, Bossuyt PM, et al. Systematic review of treatment strategies for osteochondral defects of the talar dome. Foot Ankle Clin 2003;8: 233–42.
30. Furukawa T, Eyre DR, Koide S, et al. Biochemical studies on repair cartilage resurfacing experimental defects in the rabbit knee. J Bone Joint Surg Am 1980; 62:79–89.
31. Johnson LL. Arthroscopic abrasion arthroplasty, historical and pathologic perspective: present status. Arthroscopy 1986;2:54–69.
32. Naumetz VA, Schweigel JF. Osteocartilaginous lesions of the talar dome. J Trauma 1980;20:924–7.
33. Hankemeir S, Muller EJ, Kaminski A, et al. 10-year results of bone marrow stimulating therapy in the treatment of osteochondritis dissecans of the talus. Unfallchir 2003;106(6):461–6.
34. Kumai T, Takakura Y, Higashiyama I, et al. Arthroscopic drilling for the treatment of osteochondral lesions of the talus. J Bone Joint Surg Am 1999;81:1229–35.
35. Lahm A, Erggelet C, Steinwachs M, et al. Arthroscopic management of osteochondral lesions of the talus: results of drilling and usefulness of magnetic resonance imaging before and after treatment. Arthroscopy 2000;16(3):299–304.
36. Schuman L, Struijs PA, van Dijk CN. Arthroscopic treatment for osteochondral defects of the talus. Results at follow-up at 2 to 11 years. J Bone Joint Surg Br 2002;84:364–8.
37. Takao M, Uchio Y, Kakimaru H, et al. Arthroscopic drilling with debridement of remaining cartilage for osteochondral lesions of the talar dome in unstable ankles. Am J Sports Med 2004;32(2):332–6.
38. Acevedo JI, Busch MT, Ganey TM, et al. Coaxial portals for posterior ankle arthroscopy: an anatomic study with clinical correlation on 29 patients. Arthroscopy 2000;16:836–42.
39. Giannini S, Vannini F. Operative treatment of osteochondral lesions of the talar dome: current concepts review. Foot Ankle Int 2004;25(3):168–75.
40. Hangody L, Fules P. Autologous osteochondral mosaicplasty for the treatment of full-thickness defects of weight-bearing joints: ten years of experimental and clinical experience. J Bone Joint Surg Am 2003;85(Suppl 2):25–32.
41. Bazaz R, Ferkel RD. Treatment of osteochondral lesions of the talus with autologous chondrocyte implantation. Tech Foot Ankle Surg 2004;3(1):45–52.
42. Zengerink M, Szerb I, Hangody L, et al. Current concepts: treatment of osteochondral ankle defects. Foot Ankle Clin 2006;11:331–59.
43. Gross AE, Agnidis Z, Hutchinson CR. Osteochondral defect of the talus treated with fresh osteochondral allograft transplantation. Foot Ankle Int 2001;22: 385–91.
44. Zimmer DeNovo® NT Natural Tissue graft. Warsaw, IN: Zimmer, Inc. Available at: www.zimmer.com.
45. American College of Foot and Ankle Surgeons 2012 Annual Scientific Conference San Antonio, Texas. March 1–4, 2012.

46. Kruse D, Ng A, Paden M, et al. Arthroscopic De novo NT® juvenile allograft cartilage implantation in the talus: a case presentation. J Foot Ankle Surg 2012;51: 218–21.
47. van Bergen C, Zengerink M, Blankevoort L, et al. Novel metallic implantation technique for osteochondral defects of the medial talar dome, a cadaver study. Acta Orthop 2010;81(4):495–502.
48. Jackson DW, Lalor PA, Aberman HM, et al. Spontaneous repair of full-thickness defects of articular cartilage in goat model. A preliminary study. J Bone Joint Surg Am 2001;83(1):53–64.
49. Loening AM, James IE, Levenston ME, et al. Injurious mechanical compression of bovine articular cartilage induces chondrocyte apoptosis. Arch Biochem Biophys 2000;381(2):205–12.
50. Milentijevic D, Torzilli PA. Influence of stress rate on water loss, matrix deformation and chondrocyte viability in impacted articular cartilage. J Biomech 2005;38(3): 493–502.
51. Fragomen A. Clinical case review: ankle distraction arthroplasty: MRI findings. Morrisville, PA: Small Bone Innovations, Inc. RingFix™ RAD; 2009.

Ankle Arthrodiastasis and Interpositional Ankle Exostectomy

Bryan A. Sagray, DPM, Bradley A. Levitt, DPM,
Thomas Zgonis, DPM*

KEYWORDS

- Ankle • Arthrodiastasis • External fixation • Distraction • Arthritis

KEY POINTS

- Ankle joint destructive procedures include arthrodesis and total ankle replacement.
- Ankle arthrodesis is considered by many investigators the gold standard for end-stage ankle arthrosis.
- Ankle arthrodiastasis may be considered an alternative in younger and active patient population.
- Arthrodiastasis is usually combined with an interpositional ankle exostectomy and/or ankle or calcaneal/subtalar joint correction when indicated.
- Circular external fixation is most commonly used for the ankle arthrodiastasis procedure.

INTRODUCTION

Ankle arthrosis is an uncommon pathology that affects the lower extremity, with approximately 70% comprised of a posttraumatic cause.[1] Posttraumatic ankle arthrosis often develops from a combination of factors, including direct cartilage damage and altered structural or functional integrity of joint kinematics.[2] The resulting articular damage and ankle instability is further compounded by incongruence with improper load-bearing characteristics. All of these factors ultimately accelerate the progression of ankle arthrosis.[2,3] This pathology often presents in younger and more active patient population, thus requiring joint reconstructive procedures.

Initial treatment of ankle arthrosis consists of traditional conservative measures, including but not limited to nonsteroidal anti-inflammatory medications, physical therapy, therapeutic intra-articular joint injections, shoe modification, and lifestyle

Division of Podiatric Medicine and Surgery, Department of Orthopaedic Surgery, University of Texas Health Science Center at San Antonio, 7703 Floyd Curl Drive, MSC 7776, San Antonio, TX 78229, USA
* Corresponding author.
E-mail address: zgonis@uthscsa.edu

Clin Podiatr Med Surg 29 (2012) 501–507
http://dx.doi.org/10.1016/j.cpm.2012.07.006   podiatric.theclinics.com
0891-8422/12/$ – see front matter © 2012 Elsevier Inc. All rights reserved.

changes. There are many surgical options that can be offered to patients, which generally fall into 2 groups. First are the joint destructive procedures, such as ankle arthrodesis or joint replacement. The second includes joint-sparing or reparative procedures, such as osteochondral autograft or allograft transplantation, microfracture, retrograde drilling, arthroscopic joint débridement, supramalleolar or calcaneal/subtalar joint deformity correction, and arthrodiastasis. Factors to consider in the decision-making process for any of these procedures include, but are not limited to, advancement of disease, age, health status, lifestyle, alignment, and patient expectations.

ANKLE JOINT DESTRUCTIVE PROCEDURES

Historically, arthrodesis of the ankle was considered the gold standard when conservative measures had failed to provide adequate relief. Long-term studies of ankle arthrodesis, however, demonstrate functional limitations, adjacent joint arthritis, long periods of immobilization, and a revision rate of 11% at 5 years.[4,5] Ankle joint replacement, which some literature suggests as an alternative to arthrodesis, is limited by the generally accepted notion that ideal candidates for a replacement are aged 50 to 60s, with average to low body mass index, low level of activity, good bone stock, minimal comorbidities, and minimal varus or valgus alignment.

ANKLE JOINT–SPARING PROCEDURES

Traditional surgical treatment modalities include simple ankle exostectomy, curettage, synovectomy, and/or ostechondral drilling. Recent advances in this area have allowed for new modalities to repair or salvage the ankle joint, all with differing levels of efficacy.

Cartilage transplant involves resection and replacement of the arthritic aspects of the joint with cartilage. Cartilage regeneration, a newer concept, is accomplished by stimulating the bone marrow adjacent to the defect, causing neovascularization of the subchondral bone. Such procedures include microfracture, drilling (antegrade, retrograde, and transmalleolar), and biologics (**Fig. 1**). Microfracture, usually completed arthroscopically, is when instrumentation is introduced into a portal site and driven down into the defect of the cartilage piercing the subchondral plate. This process recruits mesenchymal cells to the region, and the formation of a stable clot is vital to success of the procedure.[6] The mechanism of action behind drilling is identical to that of microfracture; however, an arthrotomy must be performed for visualization. Biologics may augment marrow-inducing techniques by serving as a scaffold for mesenchymal cells along with increasing stability of the fibrin clot.[7]

Distraction arthroplasty is based on the hypothesis that cartilage self-repairs when mechanical stress is removed.[8] In 1978, Judet and Judet[9] demonstrated in animals that distraction arthroplasty of the tibiotalar joint could produce material similar in appearance to that of normal articular cartilage. A widely accepted theory for the mechanism of action behind this process is that intermittent hydrostatic changes on a joint prevented from loading elicits cartilage repair.[10] Using a circular external fixation distraction device, off-loading of the subchondral bone and intermittent fluid pressure changes as well as minimizing neurovascular insult can be achieved.[11–13]

In 2008, Paley and colleagues[14] evaluated 32 patients who underwent typical joint-sparing techniques, including exostectomy, synovectomy, and/or corrective osteotomies, followed by application of distraction arthroplasty. Approximately 78% of their patients maintained their ankle joint range of motion and only 1 patient required subsequent arthrodesis.[14] Similar patient characteristics and reproducible results have also been cited for articular resurfacing.

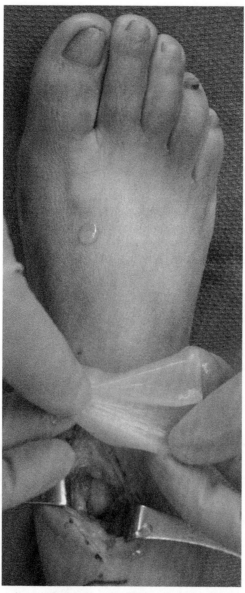

Fig. 1. Intraoperative clinical picture showing an interpositional ankle exostectomy with talar drilling and resurfacing with a biologic layer.

OPERATING TECHNIQUE

Examination begins with an in-depth review of the date and mechanism of injury as they relate to a patient's ankle pain. Knowledge of any associated soft tissue injury is also important to help estimate the amount of force impacted to the lower extremity. A thorough past medical and social history regarding tobacco and alcohol usage, support system at home, job type, and ability to maintain non–weight bearing, if indicated, are necessary for a patient's overall successful outcome.

A detailed physical examination is accompanied by plain radiographs and advanced imaging when necessary. Radiographs need to include foot, ankle, calcaneal-axial, and full-length tibia-fibula or even more proximal views according to a patient's history. These allow for assessment of gross alignment, angular deformities, nonunions, previous/current bone infection, articular incongruity, and large osteochondral lesions. The vascular and neurologic components of the examination are also critical, because this patient population may present with compromised distal perfusion or unrecognized peripheral nerve injuries. Ankle joint range of motion, mobility, and compensation influence the surgical plan as well, determining if adjacent joints require arthrodesis. The physical examination ends with weight-bearing and gait analysis to delineate any further abnormalities.

The operative technique for an isolated ankle arthrodiastasis and interpositional ankle exostectomy starts with an open ankle arthrotomy, followed by débridement of hypertrophied synovium and tibiotalar exostosis, relieving impingement.[15] Visible transchondral lesions are then addressed with the microfracture technique and talar dome resurfacing is completed with the application of a biologic layer.[15] This is followed by the application of a circular external fixation device for the final step of ankle distraction. Acute correction/distraction is usually accomplished on the operative table or gradually

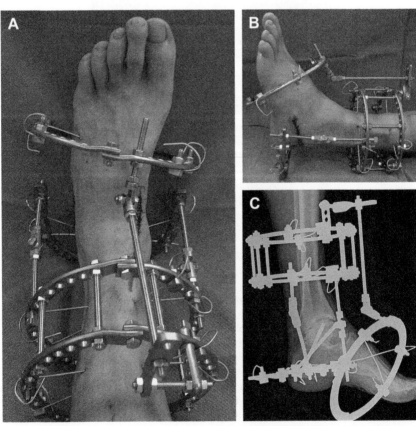

Fig. 2. Postoperative clinical (A, B) and radiographic (C) views of an ankle exostectomy and arthrodiastasis combined with a simultaneous subtalar joint arthrodesis and equinus correction in a patient with posttraumatic tibiotalocalcaneal arthrosis.

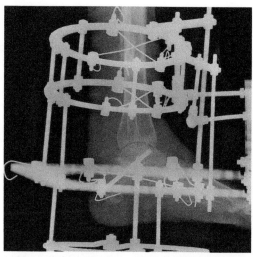

Fig. 3. Postoperative view demonstrating a combined ankle arthrodiastasis, equinus correction, and subtalar joint arthrodesis with the use of circular external fixation.

postoperatively with threaded rods and manual/distal-longitudinal traction of approximately 10 mm.[15] Postoperatively, patients are allowed to maintain a weight-bearing status or may be delayed for a short period of time if a concomitant subtalar joint arthrodesis is performed, thereby establishing the hydrostatic/distraction properties of the procedure.

The ankle arthrodiastasis and interpositional ankle exostectomy procedure may also be combined with a simultaneous subtalar joint arthrodiastasis or arthrodesis and/or calcaneal correctional osteotomy (**Figs. 2** and **3**). In addition, a supramalleolar osteotomy and/or equinus correction may be necessary in certain case scenarios with a more proximal deformity and equinus contracture.

DISCUSSION

Ankle joint arthrosis continues to be a common problem after lower extremity trauma and its treatment comprises a significant proportion of the United States total health care budget annually.[16]

Ankle arthrodiastasis has been well published in the literature and the indications continue to expand. Distraction arthroplasty may be considered before joint destructive procedures, such as arthrodesis and total ankle replacement, because it may negate the need to perform a definitive operation.[17–20] The concept of ankle joint surface or articular cartilage reconstruction is not new, but the techniques used to accomplish it are rapidly evolving. One of the most recent applications of cartilage repair advocates biologic resurfacing of articular cartilage through neovascularization.[20] This process differs from angiogenesis in that new microvascular networks are created and are able to receive perfusion, whereas angiogenesis relates to the ability to form capillary outgrowths from existing vessels.[21] The implant fulfills 2 unique criteria by providing a biologic scaffold for the native tissue to grow into, inducing neovascularization.[22]

The combination of these 2 procedures, arthrodiastasis and articular resurfacing via biologic implantation, is a new phenomenon.[23–25] The short-term results of the combined techniques seem promising; however, more detailed and controlled trials need to be performed.

SUMMARY

The surgical management of posttraumatic ankle arthrosis continues to evolve along with advances in total ankle replacement systems and locking fixation for arthrodesis. Long-term follow-up for the available surgical options and statistical data are important, with a clear need for prospective randomized clinical trials.

REFERENCES

1. Saltzman CL, Salamon ML, Blanchard GM, et al. Epidemiology of ankle arthritis: report of a consecutive series of 639 patients from a tertiary orthopaedic center. Iowa Orthop J 2005;25:44–6.
2. Robroy ML, Stewart GW, Conti SF. Posttraumatic ankle arthritis: an update on conservative and surgical management. J Orthop Sports Phys Ther 2007;37(5): 253–9.
3. Furman BD, Olson SA, Guilak F. The development of posttraumatic arthritis after articular fracture. J Orthop Trauma 2006;20:719–25.
4. SooHoo NF, Zingmond DS, Ki CY. Comparison of reoperation rates following ankle arthrodesis and total ankle arthroplasty. J Bone Joint Surg AM 2007;89:2143–9.
5. Haddad SL, Coetzee JC, Estok R, et al. Intermediate and long-term outcomes of total ankle arthroplasty and ankle arthrodesis. A systematic review of the literature. J Bone Joint Surg Am 2007;89(9):1899–905.
6. Bedi A, Feeley BT, Williams RJ 3rd. Management or articular defects of the knee. J Bone Joint Surg Am 2010;92(4):994–1009.
7. McNickle AG, Provencher MT, Cole BJ. Overview of existing cartilage repair technology. Sports Med Arthrosc Rev 2008;16:196–201.
8. van Roermund PM, Marijnissen AC, Lafeber FP. Joint distraction as an alternative for the treatment of osteoarthritis. Foot Ankle Clin 2002;7(3):515–27.
9. Judet R, Judet T. The use of a hinge distraction apparatus after arthrolysis and arthroplasty. Rev Chir Orthop Reparatrice Appar Mot 1978;64(5):2649–51.
10. Chiodo CP, McGarvey W. Joint distraction for the treatment of ankle osteoarthritis. Foot Ankle Clin 2004;9(3):541–53.
11. Marijnissen AC, van Roermund PM, van Melkebeek J, et al. Clinical benefit of joint distraction in the treatment of severe osteoarthritis of the ankle: proof of concept in an open prospective study and in a randomized controlled trial. Arthritis Rheum 2002;46(11):2893–902.
12. van Valburg AA, van Roy HL, Lafeber FP, et al. Beneficial effects of intermittent fluid pressure of low physiological magnitude on cartilage and inflammation in osteoarthritis: an in vitro study. J Rheumatol 1998;25(3):515–20.
13. Lafeber FP, Veldhuijzen JP, Vanroy JL, et al. Intermittent hydrostatic compressive forces stimulates exclusively the proteoglycan synthesis of osteoarthritic human cartilage. Br J Rheumatol 1992;31(7):437–42.
14. Paley D, Lamm BM, Purohit RM, et al. Distraction arthroplasty of the ankle—how far can you stretch the indications? Foot Ankle Clin 2008;13(3):471–84.
15. Ramanujam CL, Sagray BA, Zgonis T. Subtalar joint arthrodesis, ankle arthrodiastasis and talar dome resurfacing with the use of a collagen-glycosaminoglycan monolayer. Clin Podiatr Med Surg 2010;27(2):327–33.
16. Brown TD, Johnston RC, Saltzman CL, et al. Posttraumatic osteoarthritis: a first estimate of incidence, prevalence, and burden of disease. J Orthop Trauma 2006;20(10):739–44.
17. Labovitz JM. The role of arthrodiastasis in salvaging arthritic ankles. Foot Ankle Spec 2010;3(4):201–4.

18. Van Valburg AA, van Roermund PM, van Melkebeek AC, et al. Joint distraction in the treatment of osteoarthritis: a 2 year follow-up of the ankle. Osteoarthr Cartil 1999;7:474–9.
19. Ploemakers JJ, van Roermund PM, van Melkebeek J, et al. Prolonged clinical benefit from joint distraction in the treatment of ankle osteoarthritis. Osteoarthr Cartil 2005;13(7):582–8.
20. Berlet GC, Hyer CF, Lee TH, et al. Interpositional arthroplasty of the first MTP joint using a regenerative tissue matrix for the treatment of advanced hallux rigidus. Foot Ankle Int 2008;29(1):10–21.
21. Rucker M, Laschke MW, Junker D, et al. Angiogenic and inflammatory response to biodegradable scaffolds in dorsal skinfold chambers of mice. Biomaterials 2006;27(29):5027–38.
22. Rashid OM, Nagahashi M, Takabe K. Management of massive soft tissue defects: the use of INTEGRA® artificial skin after necrotizing soft tissue infection of the chest. J Thorac Dis 2012;4(3):331–5.
23. Ramanujam CL, Kissel S, Stewart A, et al. First metatarsophalangeal joint arthrodiastasis and biologic resurfacing with external fixation: a case report. Clin Podiatr Med Surg 2012;29(1):137–41.
24. Brigido SA, Troiano M, Schoenhaus H. Biologic resurfacing of the ankle and first metatarsophalangeal joint: case studies with a 2-year follow-up. Clin Podiatr Med Surg 2009;26(4):633–45.
25. Hyer CF, Granata JD, Berlet G, et al. Interpositional arthroplasty of the first metatarsophalangeal joint using a regenerative tissue matrix for the treatment of advanced hallux rigidus: 5-year case series follow-up. Foot Ankle Spec 2012; 5(4):249–52.

Ankle Arthrodesis: A Literature Review

Patrick A. DeHeer, DPM[a],*, Shirley M. Catoire, DPM[b],
Jessica Taulman, DPM[c], Brandon Borer, DPM[d]

KEYWORDS

- Ankle arthrodesis • Ankle arthritis • Ankle fixation • Arthrodesis

KEY POINTS

- Indications of ankle arthrodesis: pain and deformity of ankle and hindfoot.
- Approaches: anterior, lateral, mini-arthrotomy, arthroscopic.
- Fixation: 2-screw, 3-screw, or 4-screw fixation, anterior or lateral locking plates, external fixation, IM nail.
- Position: 0 to 5° of rearfoot valgus, 5 to 10° of external rotation, foot at 90° to leg.

INTRODUCTION

Ankle arthrodesis has become the mainstay surgical procedure for end-stage ankle arthritis.[1–3] There are a vast array of surgical approaches to this procedure. The end goal of any ankle arthrodesis procedure should be a well-aligned ankle joint with the foot at a 90° angle to the leg. A well-positioned ankle fusion can be very successful in alleviating pain, correcting the deformity, and restoring a functional limb.

The term arthrodesis was first described in 1878 by the Australian surgeon Eduard Alber. By the end of the 19th century, ankle and hindfoot fusions were the mainstay approach for paralytic deformities, such as polio. The first time ankle fusion was described for a malaligned ankle deformity was in the 1930s. In 1951, Charnley pioneered the "Charnley frame," which was an external fixation frame that incorporated compression arthrodesis of the ankle without bone graft. Today, joint debridement with a 3-screw or 4-screw fixation technique or arthroscopic debridement is favorable because of the low morbidity rate and higher fusion rates compared with external fixation.

INDICATIONS

Ankle arthrodesis is indicated in multiple scenarios in which there may be pain and deformity in the ankle or hindfoot. The main indication for fusion of the ankle joint is posttraumatic arthritis. Other indications for this procedure include chronic instability,

[a] 1159 West Jefferson Street, Suite 204, Franklin, IN 46131, USA; [b] 8734 Navigator Drive, Apartment 1311, Indianapolis, IN 46237, USA; [c] Resident Year 3, Community Westview Hospital, 3630 Guion Rd, Indianapolis, IN 46222, USA; [d] Resident Year 2, Community Westview Hospital, 3630 Guion Rd, Indianapolis, IN 46222, USA
* Corresponding author.
E-mail address: padeheer@gmail.com

Clin Podiatr Med Surg 29 (2012) 509–527
http://dx.doi.org/10.1016/j.cpm.2012.07.001
0891-8422/12/$ – see front matter © 2012 Elsevier Inc. All rights reserved.

rheumatoid arthritis, Charcot neuropathy with instability of the ankle joint, failed total ankle arthroplasty with implant, septic arthritis/infection of the ankle joint, avascular necrosis of the talus, and paralytic deformities when muscle tendon rebalancing is not possible.

Preoperative planning of an ankle fusion can be extensive. Before making the decision of fusing the ankle joint, the surgeon must evaluate the integrity of the surrounding joints, in particular the subtalar joint. The surgeon must take into consideration the amount of compensation that will come from the midtarsal joints, tarsal-metatarsal joints, and the subtalar joints. Wu and colleagues[4] found that sagittal plane motion for the forefoot and transverse plane motion of the rearfoot increased after an ankle joint fusion. It is recommended that preoperative radiographs include foot, ankle, and leg films. This is especially important if considering intramedullary rod fixation, as deformity of the tibia can make insertion of the nail challenging.

CONTRAINDICATIONS

Although fusion of the ankle joint may relieve pain and symptomatology for the right patient, contraindications do exist. Patients unable to be cleared for surgery secondary to medical issues, such as uncontrolled diabetes or poor nutritional status, should not be taken to surgery. Peripheral vascular status must be evaluated and the patient should be educated on the detrimental effects of tobacco use in relation to healing potential. When considering ankle fusion with internal fixation, bone infection is also a contraindication, and other forms of fixation may be warranted, specifically external fixation.[5]

SURGICAL APPROACH

Multiple surgical approaches have been described in the literature. The earliest to date was described by the Australian surgeon Charnley. He described a transverse anterior approach to the ankle joint. This approach is excellent for exposure to the talus and the lower tibia; however, it required extensive soft tissue dissection and high rate of neurovascular compromise and embarrassment.

Midline anterior approach allows great exposure to the anterior ankle joint. This incision is made just lateral to the border of the tibialis anterior tendon (**Fig. 1**). Care must be taken to avoid damaging the medial dorsal cutaneous nerve. Through this incision, the ankle joint is exposed between the tibialis anterior tendon and the extensor hallus longus tendon. The disadvantage of this incision is that it lacks exposure to the posterior ankle joint and the malleoli. The surgeon should consider this approach when the talus has been displaced medial or lateral under the tibia in the frontal plane.

A lateral approach, otherwise known as the transfibular approach, is a common technique used today. It involves a hockey stick incision over the lateral aspect of the distal one-third of the fibula, courses the sinus tarsi, and ends at the base of the fourth metatarsal. This approach should be considered when the foot is translated forward after an old pilon fracture or when the lateral malleolus must be removed. When using this approach, the surgeon must do a fibular osteotomy to access the ankle joint (**Figs. 2** and **3**). This approach is excellent to visualize the lateral ankle joint (**Fig. 4**). After completion of the ankle joint fusion, the surgeon may use the fibula as an onlay graft; however, it is not recommended to anatomically repair the fibula. Mahan and colleagues[6] report an increased incidence of delayed or nonunion when the fibula was anatomically repaired.

The medial incision begins a few centimeters above the tibial plafond and extends over the medial tibiotalar articulation continuing distally to the talonavicular joint. Care

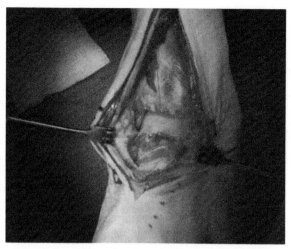

Fig. 1. Anterior approach for ankle arthrodesis. (*Courtesy of* Tornier Inc.)

is taken to identify and preserve the saphenous vein and nerve. A capsular incision is then made longitudinally and visualization of the tibiotalar joint is achieved. This medial approach gives great access to the anterior medial and posterior medial aspect of the ankle joint.

The posterior approach is unfavorable but described in the literature. It is an incision made on the posterior aspect of the leg parallel to the Achilles tendon. This technique gives poor visibility to the ankle joint and possible inadvertent risk to the subtalar joint.

The favored approach is to use a combination of the transfibular and medial ankle incisions to allow great access to the entire ankle joint.

Minimally invasive procedures, such as arthroscopic ankle fusion, have also been on the horizon. With this approach, anterior medial and anterior lateral portals are used. The cartilage is removed via curettage. Consider arthroscopy in patients with no/minimal angular deformity. The surgeon cannot correct angular deformity with arthroscopy. Bone graft can be placed in the medial and lateral gutters to aid in joint fusion. This technique is excellent for patients with rheumatoid arthritis.

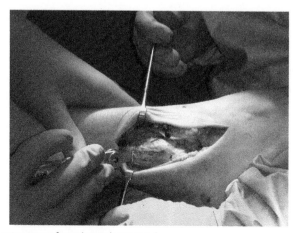

Fig. 2. Fibular osteotomy from lateral approach.

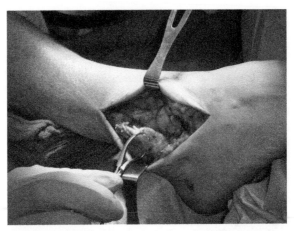

Fig. 3. Fibula being removed from operative site from lateral approach.

Winson and colleagues[7] reviewed 105 arthroscopic ankle arthrodeses. The investigators used anteromedial and anterolateral portals to access the ankle joint. Articular cartilage was removed with a soft tissue debrider and curettes. The lateral gutter was cleared enough to allow compression of the joint, and articular surfaces of the medial malleolus were removed. The investigators used a burr to remove bone until punctate bleeding was visualized in cancellous bone. Anterior tibial osteophytes were removed with the scope. Once the joint was fully prepared and cleaned, 2 percutaneous 6.5-mm screws were placed medially from the tibia to the talus. Penetration into the subtalar joint was avoided. The average time to union was 12 weeks. Nonunion occurred in 9 patients. Seven of the nonunions were successfully fused using an open arthrodesis technique. The investigators modified their postoperative protocol following a significant number of nonunions within the first 8 cases. Immobilizing the operative site for a longer period (12 weeks) postoperatively was initiated, and a decrease in the number of nonunions was seen. The investigators stated that a decreased time to union occurs in arthroscopic arthrodesis because periosteal

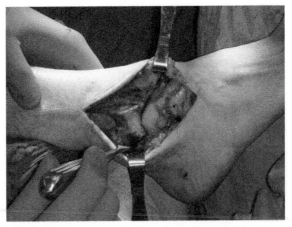

Fig. 4. Ankle exposure from lateral approach with fibula resected.

stripping is not necessary and local circulation to the bone remains intact. Nineteen percent of these patients required removal of screws because of prominence.

Miller and Myerson[8] described the mini-arthrotomy approach using 2, 1.5-cm incisions anterior medially and anterior laterally. The anterior medial incision was made just medial to the anterior tibial tendon at the level of the joint and the anterior lateral incision was made lateral to the peroneus tertius tendon at the level of the joint. With the anterior lateral incision, care must be taken to avoid the superficial peroneal nerve. A small lamina spreader was placed in the portal not being used to open the joint and allow debridement. This process was then switched to allow debridement of the other side of the joint. This approach allows limited access to the posterior aspect of the joint, but, as previously described, the limited posterior aspect of the joint that cannot be reached is inconsequential for the arthrodesis. Debridement technique is surgeon choice, but burring should be limited because of possible necrosis of the subchondral bone.

Multiple techniques have been described in the literature for preparing the ankle joint for fusion. The simplest technique is removal of cartilage from the tibia and the talus by joint resection or curettage (**Figs. 5** and **6**). Other techniques have been described, such as anterior bone grafting to facilitate fusion, joint resection with combined malleolar osteotomy, subtotal or incomplete resection of the articular cartilage, and compression arthrodesis. No matter what joint preparation the surgeon chooses, Glissan principles for successful fusion should be used. Glissan described 4 requirements for successful fusion, which include complete removal of all cartilage, accurate and close fitting or fusion surfaces, optimal position, and maintenance of bone apposition in an undisturbed fashion until fusion is achieved.[9,10] Shortening of the limb can be seen; however, if joint surfaces are prepared carefully, less than 1 cm of shortening is seen.

Optimal position of an ankle joint fusion is 0 to 5° of rearfoot valgus, 5 to 10° of external rotation (transverse plane should be in line with the normal Malleolar axis), and foot in a 90° position to the leg. Literature states that up to 5° of plantarflexion of the foot on the leg can be tolerated. Position of the fusion is the key to a successful procedure. Malalignment in the sagittal plane with ankle joint in equinus can lead to genu recurvatum. Coronal plane position is equally important with unsatisfactory results seen when the heel is in varus, leading to painful callosities to the lateral forefoot[11] and increased hindfoot symptoms.[12,13] It is important to consider equinus when positioning the foot. If a marked equinus is present during physical examination, an

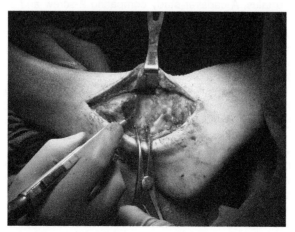

Fig. 5. Articular debridement of arthrodesis site using egg burr from lateral approach.

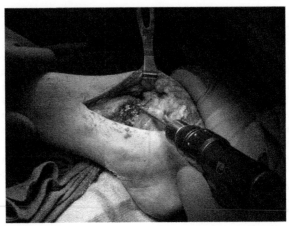

Fig. 6. Subchondral drilling of arthrodesis site using drill bit from lateral approach.

Achilles tendon or gastrocnemius lengthening may need to be performed to allow the foot to be permanently fixed at a 90° angle to the lower leg. Zwipp and colleagues[14–22] recommend performing a percutaneous lengthening of the Achilles tendon in patients with an equinus greater than 10°.

When fusing the ankle joint, it is important to keep in mind the 4 following principles for a successful fusion: (1) good alignment of the fusion with the rearfoot aligned to the leg and the forefoot to the rearfoot; (2) apposition of broad, flat, vascularized bony surfaces; (3) stable and rigid internal or external fixation; and (4) compression across the arthrodesis site.[23]

FIXATION APPROACH

Several fixation modalities have also been described in the literature ranging from bone grafting, internal fixation, external fixation, or a combination. If using screw fixation, 4.5, 6.5, or 7.3 screws are acceptable.

The 2-screw fixation technique, as described by Ogilvie-Harris and colleagues,[24] places 1 screw from the medial malleolus into the talus and 1 screw from the lateral malleolus into the talus. A cadaver study comparing 2-screw and 3-screw fixation was performed by Ogilvie-Harris and colleagues.[24] The investigators determined that the 3-screw construct gave increased compression when compared with the 2-screw construct. The 2-screw construct is not commonly used today, as other techniques have proven to be more stable and provide more compression at the arthrodesis site (**Figs. 7–9**).

The 3-screw fixation technique, as performed by Hendrickx and colleagues,[25–32] used three 4.5-mm fully threaded lag screws. The medial screw was placed anterior in the talar body. The lateral screw was placed more posterior to the medial screw into the talar body. Another 4.5-mm screw was inserted into the reduced fibula directed medially across the tibia.

In the study performed by Hendrickx and colleagues,[25] they evaluated 66 ankles with the 3-screw fixation technique performed on them with an average follow-up of 9 years. They found that in 52 ankles, the time to union was 6 weeks. In 6 ankles, the time to union was 8 weeks. Bony union took up to 12 weeks in 2 patients. One malunion and 4 nonunions were found over the course of follow-up. Good functional results were found with a high union rate using the 3-screw technique of fixation.

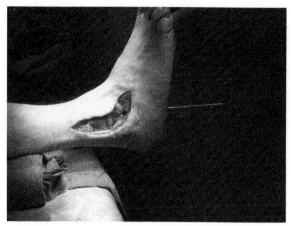

Fig. 7. Temporary fixation of ankle fusion with Steinman pin fixation.

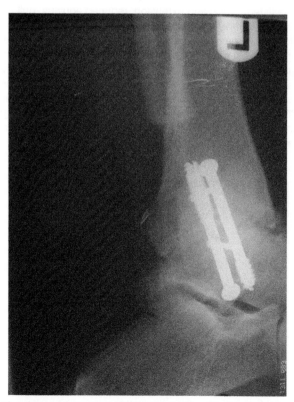

Fig. 8. Ankle arthrodesis with 2-screw fixation and onlay fibular graft lateral view.

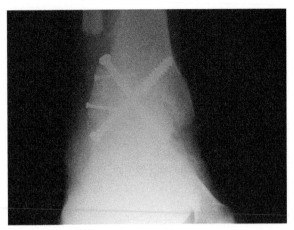

Fig. 9. Ankle arthrodesis with 2-screw fixation and onlay fibular graft anterior view.

The 3-screw configuration described by Holt and colleagues[33] involves insertion of 1 screw from the medial malleolus into the lateral body of the talus. The second screw is inserted from the lateral malleolus into the medial talar body. The third screw is placed from the posterior malleolus into the talar neck. Holt and colleagues[33] thought the most important screw was the posterior screw. This screw was considered important, because it resisted flexion and extension, reduced equinus, pulled the talus posteriorly, and provided compression across the joint surfaces (**Figs. 10–12**).

Jeng and colleagues[23] wanted to determine which of the 3 screws described by Holt and colleagues[33] provided the most initial compression at the ankle joint to determine the order for screw placement. A study was performed on 17 cadaver limbs. The investigators used film templates to evaluate contact area and pressure at the ankle joint with each screw. No difference was found between the medial, lateral, and posterior screws in total contact area, percent contact area, or pressure generated. They determined that the order of screw insertion does not affect the amount of compression achieved at the site of the arthrodesis.

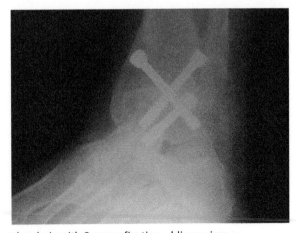

Fig. 10. Ankle arthrodesis with 3-screw fixation oblique view.

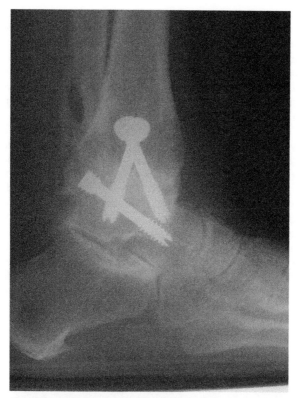

Fig. 11. Ankle arthrodesis with 3-screw fixation lateral view.

When performing the 4-screw fixation technique, as previously described by Zwipp and colleagues,[1] four 6.5-mm cancellous lag screws are used. Two screws are placed parallel from the anterior distal tibia into the talar body. The third screw is inserted 3 cm proximal to the tip of the medial malleolus through a posteromedial stab incision. The final screw is inserted from the posterolateral aspect of the distal fibula approximately

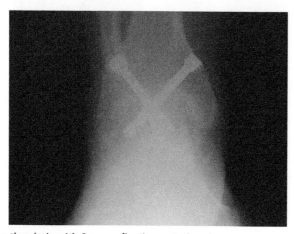

Fig. 12. Ankle arthrodesis with 3-screw fixation anterior view.

1.5 cm proximal to the lateral malleolar tip directed into the dorsal body of the talus. Fully threaded screws can be used if great bony defects or poor bone stock is present. A study was performed by Zwipp and colleagues[14] on 94 patients using the 4-screw fixation technique. These patients were followed for an average of 4.8 years, and 93 achieved union at the ankle joint. The mean American Association of Foot and Ankle Surgeons score increased from 36 to 85 following the surgery. They advocate for early active and passive range of motion (ROM) of the midtarsal and subtalar joints to have increased ROM following the procedure.

Internal bone graft with screw and staple fixation is a viable method for ankle fusion and is especially helpful in cases in which the body of the talus is not available for fusion. This method is done via the anterior approach. The ankle joint is prepared; a prism-shaped bone graft from the lower tibia is taken. While the ankle is immobilized in the neutral position, a triangular hole approximately 1.5 cm deep is made in the talus. The graft is transposed distally and fixed with screws while the ankle is fixed with compression staple on either side of the bone graft for increased stability in all planes.[34]

Anterior plating with the use of a narrow dynamic compression plate is a good method to achieve ankle fusion in many types of ankle arthropathies. Anterior plates are specifically contoured for ankle fusion with an approximate 30° proximal curve and 40° distal curve totaling a final bend of 70°.[35] Internal fixation is superior to external fixation considering clinical and biomechanical trials that have shown rigid internal fixation leading to increased rates of union and a reduced infection rate, decreased time of union, less discomfort, and earlier mobilization compared with other methods (**Fig. 13**).[36,37]

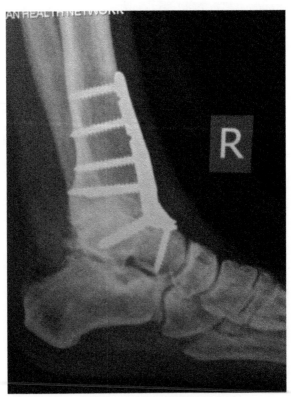

Fig. 13. Radiograph of anterior plate for ankle arthrodesis. (*Courtesy of* Tornier Inc.)

When using these plates, an anterior approach is necessary to expose the cartilaginous surfaces of the ankle mortise and allow placement of the plate. Once cartilage is removed from the ankle joint, the talus is manually compressed under the tibia and held by the anterior plate and screw construct. The first 2 screws should be placed into the talus, being careful to avoid the subtalar joint. The next screws are to be placed in the tibia and placed eccentrically to provide compression across the ankle joint. A compression screw can be place from the tibia to the talus through the proximal curve in the plate. Contouring the plate appropriately allows for compression of the tibio-talar surfaces with forward subluxation. It is also important to prevent subtalar joint penetration with the screws in the talus by using intraoperative fluoroscopy. Fixation of the midtarsal joints should be avoided initially unless pathology presents in the area or severe osteoporotic bone requires a more rigid fixation.[35]

A study by Mohamedean and colleagues[35] focused on 29 patients who had ankle arthrodesis using anteriorly placed dynamic compression plates over the course of 3 years. Twenty-two of these patients required ankle fusion owing to posttraumatic arthritis and 7 were paralytic. The average age of these patients was 24.4. Using the anterior plate, the investigators found that 100% of patients achieved fusion at an average of 12.2 weeks. The Mazur ankle score also demonstrated that 65.5% of patients had excellent results, 20.7% had good results, and 13.8% had fair results. Some complications were seen, including 4 patients with midtarsal pain and 4 patients with a long talar screw. Superficial infection was seen in 2 patients.

Locking plate technology has also been implemented in ankle arthrodesis plates both for anterior and lateral plating approaches (**Figs. 14** and **15**). Locking plates offer superior fixation to traditional plates, especially in osteopenic bone. Locking plates offer the best of both internal and external fixation. Locking plates have been the fixation method of choice for ankle arthrodesis.

The intramedullary rod can also be used to fuse the tibiotalar joint; however, this is not indicated if there is no prior subtalar joint arthritis. The rod crosses both the ankle joint and the subtalar joint, fusing both the subtalar joint and the ankle joint (**Figs. 16** and **17**). An intramedullary rod can also be beneficial for salvage procedures. A nonunion of the ankle joint with subsequent infection can be an opportunity for a permanent antibiotic impregnated intramedullary (IM) rod. Following removal of any previous hardware and adequate debridement of infected bone and soft tissue,

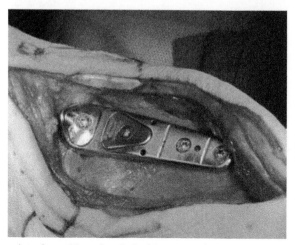

Fig. 14. Anterior plate for ankle arthrodesis. (*Courtesy of* Tornier Inc.)

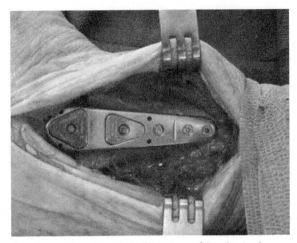

Fig. 15. Lateral plate for ankle arthrodesis. (*Courtesy of* Tornier Inc.)

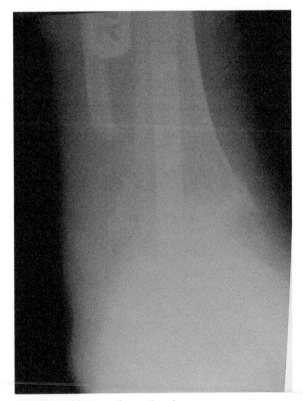

Fig. 16. Ankle arthrodesis with IM nail anterior view.

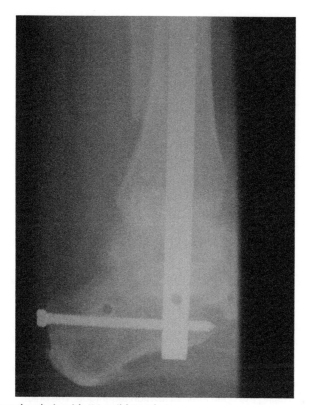

Fig. 17. Ankle arthrodesis with IM nail lateral view.

cement-coated antibiotic-impregnated IM rod can be inserted across the joint. The patient remains non–weight bearing in a cast for 8 to 10 weeks. This allows for fusion across the tibiotalar joint and local management of infection with antibiotic-impregnated cement covering the IM rod.[38]

External fixation was first described by Charnley,[39] as previously stated. He began using a single plane frame. This method of external fixation has been replaced with external fixators providing compression and controlling motion in all 3 planes. Triangular frames are now frequently used. A triangular frame designed by Calandruccio[40] is one of many devices used to fixate the tibiotalar joint.[41] This device is applied by inserting 2 pins through the talus and 2 pins through the tibia. These transverse pins are connected with the triangular frame. Other frames have been developed and transformed to provide more compression and greater pin purchase within the bone (**Figs. 18** and **19**).

The best way to achieve ankle arthrodesis is debatable. Each method of fixation has its own benefits. The arthroscopic method of fixation may have a faster time to union, less blood loss, less morbidity, a shorter hospital stay, and earlier mobilization; however, significant deformities visualized in the ankle joint are unable to be corrected with the arthroscopic method.[7] Advantages to internal fixation include ease of insertion of internal hardware; convenience to patients when compared with external fixation; similar rates of infection, delayed union, and malunion; and resistance to shear stress. External fixation can be beneficial in patients with active infection or with revisional or salvage procedures.

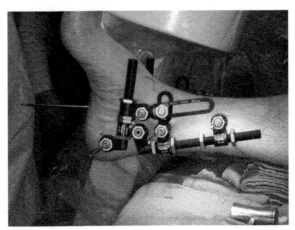

Fig. 18. External fixation for ankle fusion with Steinman pin fixation in heel lateral view.

Comparison of internal and external fixation arthrodesis was performed by Moeckel and colleagues.[37] A 95% union rate was found with internal fixation, and a 78% union rate was found with external fixation. Another study comparing fusion rates between internal and external fixation was performed by Maurer and colleagues.[42] They found a higher union with internal fixation as well, with 35 of 35 patients achieving fusion with internal fixation and 10 of 12 achieving union with external fixation.

Myerson and Quill[43] performed a study evaluating the rate to union in patients who underwent ankle arthrodesis using the arthroscopic technique and in patients who underwent fusion using the open internal fixation technique. The union rate for patients having undergone the open technique was 100% at an average for 14 weeks. A union rate of 94% in an average of 8.7 weeks was observed in the arthroscopic group.

One method used specifically for patients with long-standing rheumatoid arthritis is the Heiple technique. With this technique, the lateral malleolus is removed via a fibular osteotomy 4 to 5 cm proximal to the distal end of the tibia. The medial malleolus is excised as well. A chevron technique is used to resect the distal end of the tibia

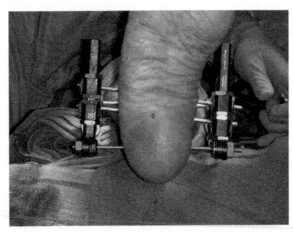

Fig. 19. External fixation for ankle fusion with Steinman pin fixation in heel plantar view.

with the point directed proximally and the arms directed distally. The talus is cut to fit into this angle of the distal tibia. The osteotomy is temporarily fixated with a Steinman pin. Staples are used to secure the osteotomy on the lateral aspect. The medial malleolus is replaced and fixed to the tibia and talus with screws. Bone graft can then be used to fill in any remaining gaps in the fusion site.[44]

Turan and Blomgren[44] performed a study to review 7 patients who underwent a chevron fusion technique for their ankle arthrodeses. Each of these patients had rheumatoid arthritis. These patients were followed an average of 44 months. Five of the 7 patients had minimal or no pain at the most recent follow-up appointment and 2 had some subtalar joint pain. All patients were satisfied with the outcome of the arthrodesis. This technique has a large contact area between the tibia and talus with the chevron cuts fitting together. By the end of immobilization following the procedure, all patients had bony fusion of the tibiotalar joint. This generally occurred by 3 months postoperatively.

POSTOPERATIVE CARE

Postoperative care can range from patient to patient. It is recommended to keep patients non–weight bearing for 8 to 12 weeks or until radiographic consolidation is visualized. A transition to partial weight bearing in a pneumatic walking boot is often started once bony trabeculation is visualized across the fusion site on radiographs. Once the patient has transitioned to regular shoe gear, modification of the shoe wear may be a necessity. Most of the time these patients require custom orthotics with a heel lift or heel cushion. They may even require a rocker bottom shoe to allow for a more normal gait pattern. Once a patient transitions into a shoe, it is beneficial to place him or her into a full-length rocker sole until the patient adapts to ambulating with a fused ankle.

COMPLICATIONS

There can be many complications for any type of major joint fusion. Overcompensation of neighboring joints is unavoidable with a large joint fusion. Gait analysis studies have shown that patients with ankle joint fusions compensate by shortening the stride length on the affected side and presumably increasing rotation at the hips and back to compensate.[45]

It is common to see arthritis in the subtalar joint (STJ), midtarsal joint, and the tarsometatarsal joint adjacent to ankle joint fusion. Bauer and Kinzl[46] reported a nonunion rate of 10% to 20%, and a postoperative infection rate of 3% to 25% following ankle joint fusion.

Zwipp and colleagues[14] reported that 16.6% of patients with an ankle fusion will have arthritis of the STJ and 11.1% of these patients will have arthritis in the talonavicular joint. The literature has also shown increased incidence of medial collateral ligament instability in the knee after an ankle fusion. One of the main reasons for an ankle arthrodesis may be significant instability and/or deformity in a neuropathic patient. It has been reported that this patient population has an increased incidence of nonunions and healing problems. In 1990, Stuart and Morrey reported a 62% complication rate and 62% reoperation rate in patients with diabetic neuropathy.[47] With any type of surgical procedure, it is importation to educate patients on the harmful effects of tobacco use. Cobb and colleagues[48] reported a 16-fold increased risk of nonunions with ankle joint fusions in smokers.

Complications other than nonunion can also arise. In many of the studies reviewed, complications often included superficial infection, deep infection surrounding hardware, prominent hardware, malalignment with fusion in varus, midtarsal pain, and long talar screws protruding into the subtalar joint.

ANKLE FUSION VERSUS ANKLE IMPLANT

With advances in technology, ankle implants have been in favor in the right patient. Total ankle arthroplasty with implantation is ideal for a patient with osteoarthritis with good ligamentous stability, reasonable anatomy, and no frontal plane deformity. Patients with rheumatoid arthritis who are not on long-term steroid use and without significant bone erosion are also good candidates for total ankle implant. Literature has reported poor outcomes of total ankle implants in young patients with posttraumatic degenerative joint disease. Total ankle implants are contraindicated with significant talar tilt, failed ankle joint fusion, significant angular deformity, and avascular necrosis of the talus.

Ankle fusion may be necessary following failure of an ankle implant. Limb length shortening is frequently a problem when converting a failed ankle arthroplasty to an ankle arthrodesis. Henricson and Rydholm[49] reviewed 13 patients with failed ankle implants who were converted to fusions. The investigators used the original incision and removed the ankle implant hardware. Following hardware removal, the bone surfaces were debrided and prepared for the Trabecular Metal Tibial Cone (Zimmer, Warsaw, IN). Once the tibial cone was inserted between the tibial and talar surfaces, the central aspect of the cone was filled with morselized bone graft. Then a retrograde IM nail was placed through the cone and screws were used to fixate the IM nail. The investigators found that after 1.4 years, 7 patients were free from pain and 4 were satisfied with the outcome with some residual pain. The other 2 patients experienced some pain with walking, particularly in the subtalar joint. The investigators concluded that using trabecular metal implants in ankle fusions after failed total ankle replacements is beneficial to restore leg length.

SUMMARY

Ankle joint arthrodesis should be considered the gold standard procedure for end-stage ankle arthritis in the appropriate patient. Incisional approach and fixation technique should be based on the patient and his or her specific needs. Arthrodesis can

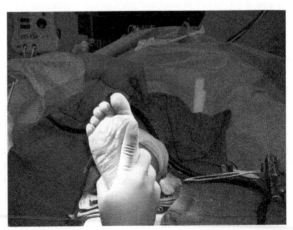

Fig. 20. Evaluation of external rotation of foot for ankle fusion using the knee cap as reference.

be achieved with adequate resection of cartilage, good compression across the fusion site, stable fixation, proper postoperative protocol, and patient compliance. It is important to remember that positioning of the ankle joint is a keystone in ankle arthrodesis (**Fig. 20**). There are complications that can arise from the ankle fusion, including the need for further surgical intervention owing to arthritis in the subtalar and midtarsal joints.

REFERENCES

1. Berkowitz MJ, Clare MP, Walling AK, et al. Salvage of failed total ankle arthroplasty with fusion using structural allograft and internal fixation. Foot Ankle Int 2011;32(5):S493–502.
2. Kleiber BD, Klein SE, McCormick JJ, et al. Radiographic analysis of wedge allograft correction of angular malalignment in ankle fusions. Foot Ankle Int 2011;32(4):380–4.
3. Jameson SS, Augustine A, James P, et al. Venous thromboembolic events following foot and ankle surgery in the English National Health Service. J Bone Joint Surg Br 2011;93(4):490–7.
4. Wu WL, Su FC, Cheng YM. Gait analysis after ankle arthrodesis. Gait Posture 2000;11:54–61.
5. Lowery NJ, Joseph AM, Burns PR. Tibiotalocalcaneal arthrodesis with the use of humeral locking plate. Clin Podiatr Med Surg 2009;26:485–92.
6. Mahan KT, Yu GV, Kalish SR. Podiatry Institute ankle fusion technique. J Am Podiatr Med Assoc 1997;87:101–16.
7. Winson IG, Robinson DE, Allen PE. Arthroscopic ankle arthrodesis. J Bone Joint Surg Br 2005;87(3):343–7.
8. Miller SD, Myerson MS. Tibiotalar arthrodesis. Foot and Ankle Clinics, vol. 1. Philadelphia: WB Saunders; 1996. p. 151–62.
9. Glissan DJ. The indications for inducing ankle joint fusion by operation with description of two successful techniques. Aust N Z J Surg 1949;19:64–71.
10. Horwitz T. The use of transfibular approach in arthrodesis of the ankle joint. Am J Surg 1942;60:550–2.
11. Mazur JM, Schwartz E, Simon SR. Ankle arthrodesis: long-term follow-up gait analysis. J Bone Joint Surg Am 1979;61:964–75.
12. Morrey BF, Wideman GP Jr. Complications and long-term results of ankle arthrodesis following trauma. J Bone Joint Surg Am 1980;62:777–84.
13. Coester LM, Saltzman CL, Leupold J, et al. Long-term results following ankle arthrodesis for post-traumatic arthritis. J Bone Joint Surg Am 2001;83:219–28.
14. Zwipp H, Rammelt S, Endres T, et al. High union rates and function scores at midterm follow-up with ankle arthrodesis using a four screw technique. Clin Orthop Relat Res 2010;468(4):958–68.
15. Dreher T, Hagmann S, Wenz W. Reconstruction of multiplanar deformity of the hindfoot and midfoot with internal fixation techniques. Foot Ankle Clin 2009; 14(3):489–531. Review.
16. Bibbo C, Patel DV, Haskell MD. Recombinant bone morphogenetic protein-2 (rhBMP-2) in high-risk ankle and hindfoot fusions. Foot Ankle Int 2009;30(7):597–603.
17. Carmont MR, Tomlinson JE, Blundell C, et al. Variability of joint communications in the foot and ankle demonstrated by contrast enhanced diagnostic injections. Foot Ankle Int 2009;30(5):439–42.
18. Rochman R, Jackson Hutson J, Alade O. Tibiocalcaneal arthrodesis using the Ilizarov technique in the presence of bone loss and infection of the talus. Foot Ankle Int 2008;29(10):1001–8.

19. SooHoo NF, Zingmond DS, Ko CY. Comparison of reoperation rates following ankle arthrodesis and total ankle arthroplasty. J Bone Joint Surg Am 2007; 89(10):2143–9.
20. Tang KL, Li QH, Chen GX, et al. Arthroscopically assisted ankle fusion in patients with end-stage tuberculosis. Arthroscopy 2007;23(9):919–22.
21. Bluman EM, Myerson MS. Stage IV posterior tibial tendon rupture. Foot Ankle Clin 2007;12(2):341–62 viii. Review.
22. Fabrin J, Larsen K, Holstein PE. Arthrodesis with external fixation in the unstable or misaligned Charcot ankle in patients with diabetes mellitus. Int J Low Extrem Wounds 2007;6(2):102–7.
23. Jeng CL, Baumbach SF, Campbell J, et al. Comparison of initial compression of the medial, lateral, and posterior screws in an ankle fusion construct. Foot Ankle Int 2011;32:71–6.
24. Ogilvie-Harris DJ, Fitsialos D, Hedman TP. Arthrodesis of the ankle. A comparison of two versus three screw fixation in a crossed configuration. Clin Orthop Relat Res 1994;304:195–9.
25. Hendrickx RP, Kerkhoffs GM, Stufkens SA, et al. Ankle fusion using a 2-incision, 3-screw technique. Oper Orthop Traumatol 2011;23(2):131–40. http://dx.doi.org/10.1007/s00064-011-0015-0.
26. DeCarbo WT, Granata AM, Berlet GC, et al. Salvage of severe ankle varus deformity with soft tissue and bone rebalancing. Foot Ankle Spec 2011;4(2):82–5.
27. Maskill MP, Maskill JD, Pomeroy GC. Surgical management and treatment algorithm for the subtle cavovarus foot. Foot Ankle Int 2010;31(12):1057–63.
28. Jones C, Abbassian A, Trompeter A, et al. Driving a modified car: a simple but unexploited adjunct in the management of patient with ankle pain. Foot Ankle Surg 2010;16(4):170–3.
29. Akra GA, Middleton A, Adedapo AO, et al. Outcome of ankle arthrodesis using a transfibular approach. J Foot Ankle Surg 2010;49(6):508–12.
30. Haaker R, Kohja EY, Wojciechowski M, et al. Tibo-talo-calcaneal arthrodesis by a retrograde intramedullary nail. Ortop Traumatol Rehabil 2010;12(3):245–9.
31. Tsailas PG, Wiedel JD. Arthrodesis of the ankle and subtalar joints in patients with haemophilic arthropathy. Haemophilia 2010;16(5):822–31.
32. Kanakaris NK, Mallina R, Calori GM, et al. Use of bone morphogenetic proteins in arthrodesis: clinical results. Injury 2009;40(Suppl 3):S62–6.
33. Holt ES, Hansen ST, Mayo KA, et al. Ankle arthrodesis using internal screw fixation. Clin Orthop Relat Res 1991;268:21–8.
34. Takakura Y, Tanaka Y, Sugimoto K, et al. Long term results of arthrodesis for osteoarthritis of the ankle. Clin Orthop Relat Res 1999;361:178–85.
35. Mohamedean A, Said HG, El-Sharkawi M, et al. Technique and short-term results of ankle arthrodesis using anterior plating. Int Orthop 2010;34:833–7.
36. Sohm MP, Benjamin JB, Harrison J, et al. A biomechanical evaluation of three forms of internal fixation used in ankle arthrodesis. Foot Ankle Int 1994;15:297–300.
37. Moeckel BH, Patterson BM, Inglis AE, et al. Ankle arthrodesis: a comparison of internal fixation and external fixator. Clin Orthop 1991;268:78–83.
38. Woods JB, Lowery NJ, Burns PR. Permanent antibiotic impregnated intramedullary nail in diabetic limb salvage: a case report and literature review. Diabet Foot Ankle 2012;3:11908.
39. Charnley J. Compression arthrodesis of the ankle and shoulder. J Bone Joint Surg Br 1951;33:180–91.
40. Williams JE Jr, Marcinko D, Lazerson A, et al. The Calandruccio triangular compression device: a schematic introduction. J Am Podiatry Assoc 1983;73:536–9.

41. Thordarson DB, Markolf KL, Cracchiolo A. External fixation in arthrodesis of the ankle. A biomechanical study comparing a unilateral frame with a modified transfixion frame. J Bone Joint Surg Am 1994;76:1541–4.

42. Maurer RC, Cimino WR, Cox CV, et al. Transarticular cross-screw fixation. A technique of ankle arthrodesis. Clin Orthop Relat Res 1991;(368):56–64.

43. Myerson MS, Quill G. Ankle arthrodesis. A comparison of an arthroscopic and an open method of treatment. Clin Orthop Relat Res 1991;268:84–95.

44. Turan I, Blomgren G. Ankle arthrodesis by the Heiple technique in rheumatoid arthritis. J Foot Surg 1991;30(2):143–6.

45. Cooke PH, Jones IT. Arthrosopic ankle arthrodesis. Tech Foot Ankle Surg 2007; 6(4):210–7.

46. Bauer G, Kinzl L. Arthrodesis of the ankle joint. Orthopade 1996;25(2):158–65.

47. Stuart M, Morrey B. Arthrodesis of the diabetic neuropathic ankle joint. Clin Orthop 1990;253:209–11.

48. Cobb T, Gabrielsen T, Cambell D. Cigarette smoking and nonunion after ankle arthrodesis. Foot Ankle 1994;15:581.

49. Henricson A, Rydholm U. Use of a trabecular metal implant in ankle arthrodesis after failed total ankle replacement. Acta Orthopaedica 2010;81(6):747–9.

Tibiotalocalcaneal Arthrodesis

Jesse B. Burks, DPM, MS, FACFAS

KEYWORDS

- Tibiotalocalcaneal arthrodesis (TTCA) • Ankle arthrodesis • Subtalar arthrodesis
- Pantalar arthrodesis • Ankle arthrosis • Subtalar arthrosis • Charcot arthropathy
- Limb salvage

KEY POINTS

- Tibitalocalcaneal arthrodesis (TTCA) can be an effective procedure to reduce pain.
- TTCA is a procedure that traditionally has a high complication rate.
- Intra-operative technique, anatomic positioning of the foot/ankle, and strict post-operative maintainance can significantly reduce complications.

INTRODUCTION

This author's personal patient care experience with tibiotalocalcaneal arthrodesis (TTCA) has been mixed at best. On one hand, a severely deformed, arthritic hindfoot and ankle can improve significantly with this type of arthrodesis. It can dramatically reduce pain, restore a more normal semblance of gait, and markedly improve someone's life. On the other hand, however, intraoperative or postoperative complications can lead to a worsening of all of the above and extend to loss of both life and limb. This is not to insinuate that this is a poor procedure. Rather, it is a procedure that has found a lesser role in my personal surgical practice. Although it still can afford benefits, bracing, appropriate pain management, ankle replacement, tibial realignment, hindfoot realignment, and isolated ankle or hindfoot fusions seemed to have slowly replaced this end-stage procedure more and more.[1–4]

Combined ankle and subtalar arthrodesis is a worthwhile procedure, but excellent patient selection and preparation are paramount to success. In retrospect, some of my own surgical failures were not so much related to inferior surgical technique as they were to inferior patient education with regard to expectations. This article provides only one author's experience with this surgery and each reader is urged to consider what works best in his or her surgical hands. Naturally, this is a large topic to which this article can only provide a cursory introduction. Many of the articles in this Clinics edition overlap on certain topics and the reader should find numerous, valuable, and diverse opinions throughout. This article is not intended to provide a complete review of the history or outcomes of this particular procedure. It is, rather, intended to give one surgeon's opinion and experience with the TTCA.

OrthoSurgeons, #5 Street, Vincent Circle, Suite 410, Little Rock, AR 72205, USA
E-mail address: jesse.burks@orthosurgeons.com

Clin Podiatr Med Surg 29 (2012) 529–545
http://dx.doi.org/10.1016/j.cpm.2012.08.002
0891-8422/12/$ – see front matter © 2012 Elsevier Inc. All rights reserved.

INDICATIONS
Posttraumatic Arthrosis

There are several conditions that can potentially benefit from a TTCA. **Fig. 1** illustrates a typical posttraumatic joint years after injury. Despite adequately performed open reduction and internal fixation (ORIF), many of these joints can slowly progress to this degenerative stage. Naturally, there is an even higher necessity for later fusion in the joint that is not repaired. Posttraumatic arthosis is, in the author's experience, the most common reason necessitating fusion.

Posterior Tibial Dysfunction

Whether injury to the posterior tibial tendon is acute or chronic, attenuation of the structure allows for progression of the foot into a valgus position. Although sudden onset of a valgus deformity will not immediately alter position of the ankle, chronic valgus will eventually cause attenuation of the medial lagamentous structures and allow progressive subluxation of the talocrural joint. In long-standing, severe pes planus, arthrodesis of this joint may be required.

Avascular Necrosis

Numerous conditions can contribute to loss of blood supply to the talus. The avascular necrosis (AVN) form of joint destruction is exceptionally challenging to the foot and ankle surgeon. Loss of bone, poor blood supply, and decreased bone density (and quality) can affect not only the form of fixation used but also dramatically increase the possibility of nonunion. Pagenstert and colleagues[5] reported an almost 90% rate of nonunion when a similar procedure was performed on patients with a history of talar AVN. Not only does AVN preclude use of an ankle replacement, but the diminished bone quality can increase operating room time and postoperative recovery. In this surgeon's own practice, any history of AVN often requires a 50% increase in

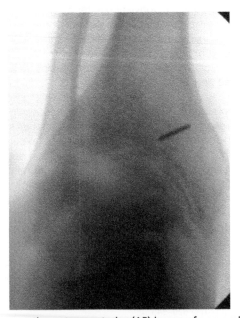

Fig. 1. Immediate preoperative anteroposterior (AP) image of a severely degenerated ankle and hindfoot secondary to previous fracture. Note prior hardware removal.

the non–weight-bearing (NWB) and immobilization period compared with patients without a history of AVN.

Rheumatoid Arthritis

Rheumatoid arthritis can be severely debilitating when affecting any portion of the lower extremity, but it is much more easily dealt with in the forefoot. Joint destruction of the hindfoot and/or ankle that requires fusion can be challenging given bone quality, treatment medications (ie, prednisone and immunosuppressive therapies), and involvement of other joints that make it difficult to remain NWB. The author has found in his practice that this group of patients seems more prone to progressive loss of postoperative position and has a higher rate of surgical revision or need for continued bracing even after reconstruction.

Diabetic Neuropathic Osteoarthropathy (Charcot)

Although this patient population may not typically present with severe pain, this a is a condition that is at the very least life-altering and at the very worst limb or life-threatening. Given that Charcot is most common in a patient population that is already at high risk, a successful TTCA in the diabetic patient can be achieved but must be coupled with aggressive management of comorbidities. This author has found that a lengthy discussion concerning realistic expectations following a successful surgery and even discussion of amputation are in order before this procedure is performed.

Failed Total Ankle Replacement Salvage

Total ankle replacement (TAR) is slowly becoming an increasingly used treatment for severe ankle degeneration. Unfortunately, in the cases that require salvage, such as infection and subsidence, TTCA is often the only choice. These cases carry higher rates of postoperative complications not only because they are revision cases but also because they usually require significant bone grafting as well. Even autogenous grafting can still be difficult to heal or prone to fixation failure (**Fig. 2**).

PREOPERATIVE CONSIDERATIONS

There are numerous preoperative factors that can affect a surgical outcome. The following is only a selection of the more common ones that can be addressed presurgically. The more factors that are addressed before surgery, the less likely the patient, and the surgeon, will be unhappy with the surgical outcome.

Psychological Preparedness

Is the patient really ready for this procedure? It is a basic question, but an extremely important one. The patient needs, first, to understand the lengthy healing period and also respect the fact that an estimated 12-week healing period is just that: "estimated." In a sense, the surgeon's role after the procedure is not just to manage the patient with regard to pain, infection, and wound and bone healing, but to also act as both a teacher and a supporter. It is best to explain set backs to the patient and provide reasons for the set backs and how they need to be dealt with.

Activity changes will also need to be discussed. Because most patients who reach the stage of requiring a TTCA have usually been limited, this author tries to counsel the patient that although the pain and/or deformity should be reduced following the procedure, there will still be significant limitations in what he or she can do. Bracing may still be needed. Shoe modifications may be needed. In those patients who still have some degree of hindfoot and ankle motion, gait changes following fusion should be

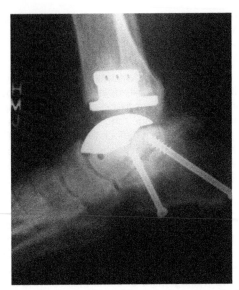

Fig. 2. Lateral view of a failed total ankle. Although the author feels total ankle replacement is a viable option in many patients, the talar component displaced distally and caused progressive pain and loss of implant motion.

discussed. Also, this author, and others,[6] have found that it is reasonable for most of these patients to require some form of long-term pain management even with a successful outcome.

Management of Comorbidities

This topic could be an entire book in and of itself. Any chronic disease that affects healing needs to be optimized. Adequate glucose control, preoperative anemia, obesity, and smoking are just a few of the issues that dramatically affect the perioperative period. It is imperative that the surgeon work closely with the patient's primary health care provider and/or hospitalist to anticipate and address these issues early. In fact, in the high-risk population, a long period in a rehabilitation facility may be needed to closely monitor not only patient therapy and compliance, but also manage other health conditions.

Discussion of Complications

Complications are difficult to discuss for both the patient and the surgeon. The TTCA is a time-tested procedure, but it carries a high chance of complications.[7] Granted, the complications can be mild, such as chronic swelling and pain, but they can also be more severe, such as infection and nonunion[5,6,8] or malunion. In many regards to TTCA it is not so much a matter of "if" but "when." Anecdotally, this author has found in practice more than half of patients with TTCA experience some form of complication.

SURGICAL TECHNIQUE

There are numerous technique modifications that have been advocated for this procedure. Most of them focus on the specific method of internal, external, or combination

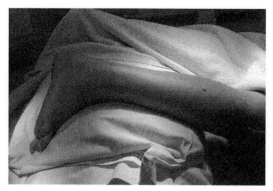

Fig. 3. Alternate prone positioning for intramedullary (IM) nail fixation.

fixation. This section, in conjunction with the associated surgical photographs, help illustrate one method only.

Positioning

Patient positioning can be varied. In certain instances, such as use of certain intramedullary locking nails, a prone position may be needed (**Fig. 3**). The author has found this to be more difficult to appropriately position the foot in the transverse plane. This may be related to the inability to visualize the patella intraoperatively. Supine seems to be the easiest to facilitate proper fixation in all 3 cardinal planes.

Incision

A lateral incision affords the surgeon complete exposure of the ankle and subtalar joints. This author usually curves the distal aspect of the incision toward the sinus tarsi

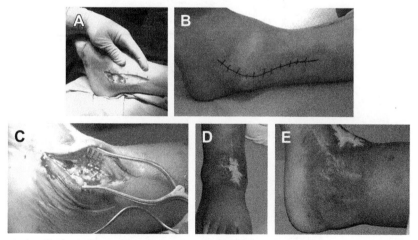

Fig. 4. (*A, B*) These figures illustrate the author's typical approach for a patient requiring both ankle and subtalar arthrodesis. In most cases, the incision is similar to that for an ankle arthrodesis, but extended slightly more distally and curved distally as well. (*C*) Alternately, a medial approach can be used. In this instance the antero-medial incision facilitated removal of a medially displaced implant. (*D, E*) Illustrates multiple scars from prior ORIF's and failed total ankle replacement. Many patients who require a TTC arthrodesis have had numerous surgeries and soft tissue healing can be a significant postoperative concern.

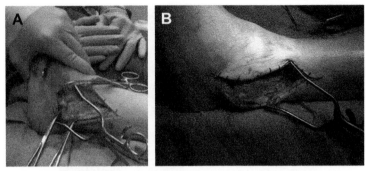

Fig. 5. (*A, B*) Exposed fibula. Some surgeons choose to use the fibula as an onlay graft later-ally. This surgeon uses the fibula as an autogenous graft to preserve limb length as much as possible.

and this allows access to all facets of the talocalcaneal joint. There are no significant structures that are prone to injury when using this incision (**Fig. 4**A, B).

Occasionally, a medial or anteromedial approach is needed (**Fig. 4**C). Except in cases in which the entire talus may be removed, this incision alone will require a secondary incision for exposure of the subtalar joint. Incision planning may need to be modified because of multiple previous surgeries. **Fig. 4**D and E show prior

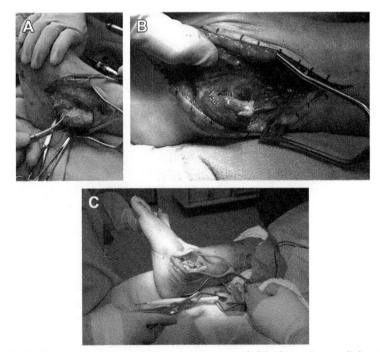

Fig. 6. (*A, B*) Fibular osteotomy complete. Joints exposed. (*C*) Alternative medial malleollar osteotomy. Of course, this does not provide exposure to the subtalar joint. In this case, the talus was removed and used as a large autogenous graft.

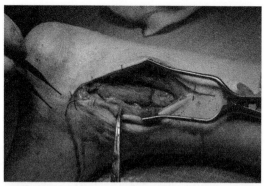

Fig. 7. Fibular exposure from a prone position.

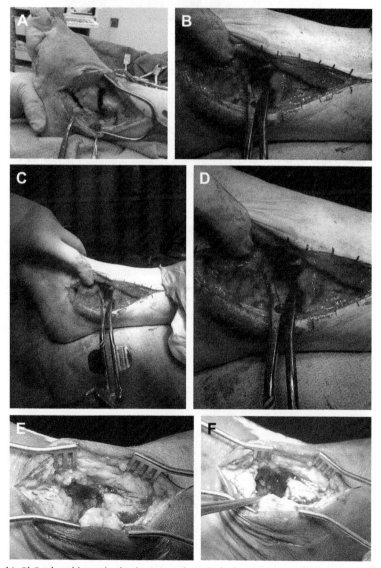

Fig. 8. (*A–D*) Both ankle and subtalar joints denuded of cartilage. Significant deformity may require more bone resection, which can require grafting to preserve limb length. (*E, F*) Joint preparation from a medial approach.

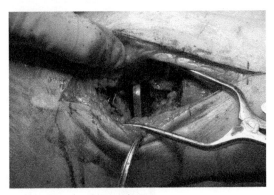

Fig. 9. Exposure of a failed total ankle implant.

incisions from ORIF, TAR, and complicated incision and drainage procedures with removal of infected bone.

Exposure of the fibula requires very little dissection and the osteotomy can be achieved with a power saw or with an osteotome and mallet. (The only structures prone to injury are the peroneal tendons, which are easily retracted.) In most cases, prior distal fibular fracture results in sclerotic bone and use of hand instruments is not practical (**Figs. 5**, **6**A, B and **7**). Again, a medial approach is not as common, but is definitely at the disposal of the surgeon (**Fig. 6**C).

Joint Preparation

Numerous surgeons have advocated different methods of joint preparation. In the end, one of the primary goals is adequate alignment of the foot in all 3 planes. Frequently, sclerosis and adaptive deformities require realignment. Because of this, the author has rarely found that curettage or minimal resection techniques are useful. The ability to change the alignment almost necessitates at least some appreciable bone resection. This may be done with use of a power saw, osteotomes, or rotary burr. Care should be taken to avoid overheating of whatever power equipment is used. TTCA is fraught with complications, and necrosis secondary to overheating of instrumentation is one that can almost surely be avoided (**Fig. 8**).

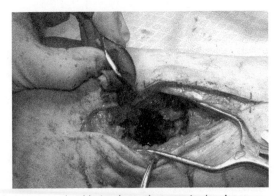

Fig. 10. Even with newer total ankle implants that require less bone removal, at least some bone loss must be surgically addressed when converted to an arthrodesis.

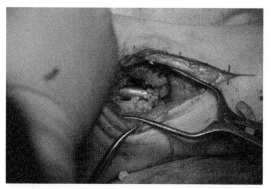

Fig. 11. Lateral view following implant removal.

Grafting

Autogeneic or allogeneic grafting is often required in TTCA. This is not only because of substantial limb length disturbance from preoperative or intraoperative issues, but also to aid in realignment of the hindfoot/ankle complex. Although iliac crest graft is

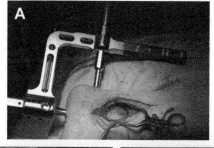

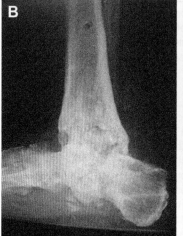

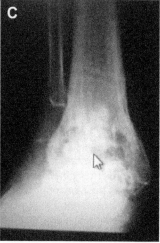

Fig. 12. (A) Lateral view with autograft in place. This graft was harvested during reaming of the medullary canal for nail insertion. (B) Final lateral radiograph of the patient from **Fig. 3** on. Naturally some limb length discrepancy occurred from loss of graft height, but this has been easily accommodated with modification to the patient's sole. (C) Final AP radiograph.

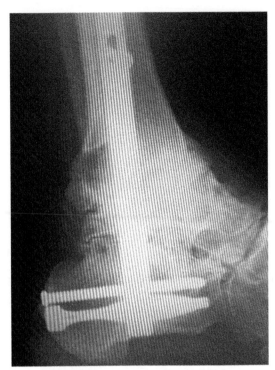

Fig. 13. Long-term radiograph following IM nail arthrodesis. This author has feels a partial subtalar nonunion is rarely symptomatic with this type of rigid fixation.

readily available, this author typically uses the distal portion of the fibula as a graft. It is readily available and provides a large amount of both cortical and cancellous bone. **Figs. 9–17** show the significant loss of one bone following failed TAR and the need for extensive grafting following implant removal. Final radiographs are also included. Although some shortening was inevitable, the patients had acceptable outcomes and limb length issues were mild and easily addressed via shoe modifications.

Foot Position

In general, the foot is placed slightly abducted from the midline of the tibia in the transverse plane. (A strict ankle arthrodesis or a TCCA patient will often benefit from a rocker bottom modification to his or her shoe. Otherwise, the normal gait pattern will become increasingly externally rotated.) Too much internal or external rotation will adversely affect the more proximal joints. In the frontal plane, up to 5° of valgus is considered acceptable. A varus position, or greater than 5° of valgus, had the same adverse affect on gait and the knee and hip. Finally, sagittal plane reduction is very important. Dorsiflexion of the foot will most likely result in the knee now fully extending during gait. The elevated forefoot is compensated by keeping the knee bent during ambulation. A slightly plantarflexed foot is more readily accommodated with a slight heel lift or similar orthotic modification; however, too much plantarflexion will force the knee into hyperextension during ambulation.[8] Mendicino and colleagues[9] provide an excellent article discussing optimal position of the rearfoot and ankle.

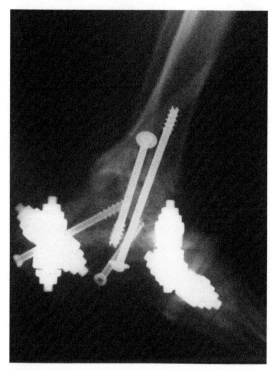

Fig. 14. Another patient, early postoperative lateral view, showing athrodesis following removal of a total ankle. Unilateral fixator was used as well.

Fixation

There are an infinite number of fixation methods that have been advocated and the references in this article are not exhaustive. The most preferred seem to have been either a locking plate modification[10,11] or an intramedullary nail construct.[12–14] This author has found that a combination of both internal and external fixation has afforded a secure form of fixation with significant compression across the arthrodesis sight **Fig. 18**.

Closure

Closure is based on the surgeon's preference, but a drain is almost always used. Otherwise, this author has found an increased incidence of dehiscence postoperatively, secondary to large hematoma formations. Especially given the bone resection that may be required, significant bleeding/drainage is the norm rather than the exception.

POSTOPERATIVE CONSIDERATIONS
Compliance

A strict NWB period during recovery is essential. Even minimal disturbance of fixation, no matter how stable the internal or external construct, can cause failure of the union. Factors that should be evaluated when considering options for the patient remaining NWB include size, upper body strength, and overall understanding of NWB importance.

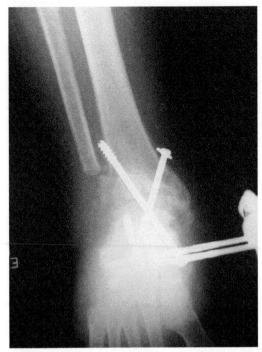

Fig. 15. Another patient, early postoperative AP view, showing athrodesis following removal of a total ankle. Unilateral fixator was used as well.

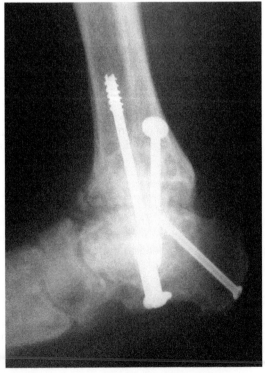

Fig. 16. Final lateral radiograph of the patient from **Figs. 14** and **15**.

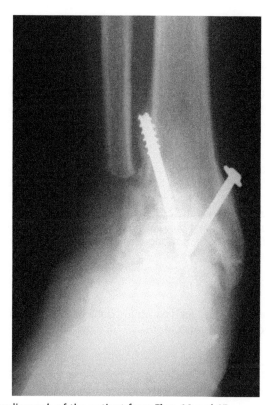

Fig. 17. Final AP radiograph of the patient from **Figs. 14** and **15**.

Occasionally noncompliance is not so much from a blatant disregard as it is a lack of understanding or a simple inability to do so.

Pain Management

Simply put, this author has found that most patients that require a TTCA will never be "pain free." Although his or her pain may be improved, it is rarely gone completely.

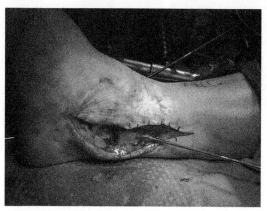

Fig. 18. Temporary fixation for cannulated screw fixation. Appropriate fixation in all 3 planes is vital to approximate normal function of the limb.

Gain changes and stress on adjacent joints (and subsequent arthrosis of those joints) still cause some level of discomfort. This level of pain may or may not require use of nonsteroidal anti-inflammatory medication or even narcotic medication. It is not uncommon that TCCA patients required use of pain medication before surgery, so this author has rarely found these patients require no medication at all. If a patient has been on long-term, but well-controlled pain medication before the surgery, it is best to have him or her evaluated before surgery by a pain specialist. Many surgeons agree that a salvage procedure such as this does not eliminate pain, but it can improve the pain.

Edema

This author has found that immediate postoperative edema is not unusual compared with other reconstructive procedures, but chronic edema is almost always present and rarely subsides completely. This should be explained to the patient. Extensive surgical dissection, bony growth required for the healing of 2 joints, and the loss of ankle motion all contribute to this. Not only will control of immediate postoperative edema facilitate closure of the incisions, but long-term control is often required with compression stockings.

COMPLICATIONS

Although minor complications, such as wound dehiscence, are common, other more serious complications can also occur.

Infection

Infection is one of the most devastating complications following TTCA. Soft tissue infections must be dealt with aggressively, as deep space infections and those

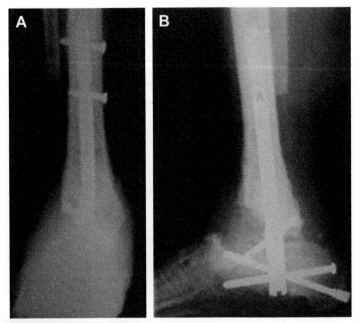

Fig. 19. (A, B) Lateral and AP views of a TTC arthrodesis with IM nail fixation. Note the lucency anteriorly. This area was cultured and osteomyelitis was confirmed.

involving bone become much more complicated and can threaten life and limb. Often bony involvement requires valiant efforts to salvage the surgery.[14–16] Jehan and colleagues[17] described, in an extensive review of the literature, an amputation rate of 1.5% in 659 procedures performed on 631 patients (**Fig. 19**).

Nonunion

The numerous variations in both internal and external fixation provide evidence that surgeons are always searching for ways to decrease the rates of failed fusions in this particular procedure. In this procedure, however, some patients remain stable and pain free despite poor radiographic union (**Fig. 20**).

Malunion

Position of the ankle and hindfoot are extremely important.[9,10] Successful fusion can be achieved, but if it is not coupled with good alignment, the patient may not benefit

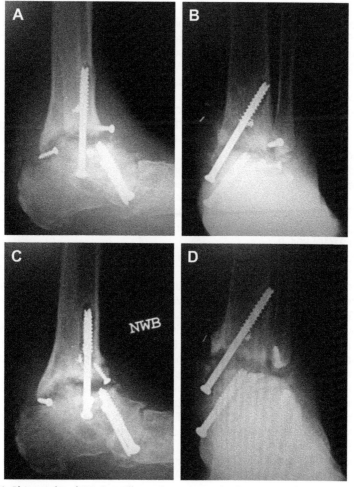

Fig. 20. (*A–D*) Lateral and AP views illustrating progressive loosening of the remaining hardware. Patient progressed to a septic nonunion.

from the procedure. Malalignment can place undue stress on adjacent joints and causes these joints to degenerate. Strict immobilization during the recovery period is important because the prolonged healing period can lead to slow deformation of the alignment if the patient bears weight prematurely.

SUMMARY

In summary, TTCA is a worthwhile procedure that can provide significant reduction in pain to appropriate patients. However, the postoperative period is not without significant and numerous obstacles that the surgeon must navigate to ensure patient recovery and a successful outcome. Although this surgeon has found the end results to be mixed, in a specific patient population it can provide tremendous benefit to the patient.

REFERENCES

1. Kim C, Catanzariti AR, Mendicino RW. Tibiotalocalcaneal arthrodesis for salvage of severe ankle degeneration. Clin Podiatr Med Surg 2009;26(2):283–302.
2. Van Roermund PM, Marijnissen AC, Lafeber FP. Joint distraction as an alternative for the treatment of osteoarthritis. Foot Ankle Clin 2002;7(3):515–27.
3. Marijnissen AC, Van Roermund PM, Van Melkebeek J, et al. Clinical benefit of joint distraction in the treatment of severe osteoarthritis of the ankle: proof of concept in an open prospective study and in a randomized controlled study. Arthritis Rheum 2002;46(11):2893–902.
4. Gould JS, Alvine FG, Mann RA, et al. Total ankle replacement: a surgical discussion. Part I. Replacement systems, indications, and contraindications. Am J Orthop 2000;29(8):604–9.
5. Pagenstert G, Knupp M, Valderrabano V, et al. Realignment surgery for valgus ankle osteoarthritis. Oper Orthop Traumatol 2009;21(1):77–87.
6. Frey C, Halikus NM, Vu-Rose T, et al. A review of ankle arthrodesis: predisposing factors to nonunion. Foot Ankle Int 1994;15(11):581–4.
7. Chou LB, Mann RA, Yaszay B, et al. Tibiotalocalcaneal arthrodesis. Foot Ankle Int 2000;21(10):804–8.
8. Cooper PS. Complications of ankle and tibiotalocalcaneal arthrodesis. Clin Orthop Relat Res 2001;(391):33–44.
9. Mendicino RW, Lamm BM, Catanzariti AR, et al. Realignment arthrodesis of the rearfoot and ankle: a comprehensive evaluation. J Am Podiatr Med Assoc 2005;95(1):60–71.
10. Buck P, Morrey B, Chao EY. The optimum position of arthrodesis of the ankle: a gait study of the knee and ankle. J Bone Joint Surg Am 1987;69(7):1052–62.
11. Ahmad J, Pour AE, Raikin SM. The modified use of a proximal humeral locking plate for tibiotalocalcaneal arthrodesis. Foot Ankle Int 2007;28:977–83.
12. DiDomenico LA, Wargo_Dorsey M. Tibiotalocalcaneal arthrodesis using a femoral locking plate. J Foot Ankle Surg 2012;51(1):128–32.
13. Goebel M, Gerdesmeyer K, Muckley T, et al. Retrograde intramedullary nailing in tibiotalocalcaneal arthrodesis: a short term, prospective study. J Foot Ankle Surg 2006;45(2):98–106.
14. Bibbo C. Treatment of the infected extended ankle arthrodesis after tibiotalocalcaneal retrograde nailing. Tech Foot Ankle Surg 2002;1:74–86.
15. Bibbo C, Lee S, Anderson RB, et al. Limb salvage: the infected retrograde tibiotalocalcaneal intramedullary nail. Foot Ankle Int 2003;24(5):420–5.

16. Mendicino RW, Bowers CA, Catanzariti AR. Antibiotic coated intramedullary rod. J Foot Ankle Surg 2008;48(2):104–10.
17. Jehan S, Shakeel M, Bing AJ, et al. The success of tibiotalocalcaneal arthrodesis with intramedullary nailing: a systematic review of the literature. Acta Orthop Belg 2011;77(5):644–51.

Total Ankle Replacement
A Historical Perspective

Benjamin D. Overley Jr, DPM

KEYWORDS

- Ankle • Replacement • Design • Prosthesis • Arthritis • Implant

KEY POINTS

- Ankle replacements were a failure in the early days of implantation.
- These failures were the impetus for new designs.
- Understanding the biomechanics and anatomy of the ankle improved the latest generation of ankle replacement implants.
- The latest generation of ankle replacements has shown increasingly positive results.
- Total ankle replacement is a viable option for certain patients with end stage ankle arthritis.

INTRODUCTION

Total ankle replacement was first attempted in the early 1970s as an alternative to ankle arthrodesis.[1–12] This procedure gave surgeons the opportunity to provide or preserve ankle motion for patients with end-stage ankle arthritis or posttraumatic arthritis (**Figs. 1** and **2**). During the 1970s, the devices that were available for ankle replacement implantation were widely criticized. This was primarily due to very poor patient outcomes with regard to the initial wave of implants that were available on the market.[1,3–5,7,8,13,14] At times, this resulted in catastrophic failures with regard to the procedure.[1,8,9,15] It was not until the 1980s and 1990s that interest was renewed as new designs that addressed the shortcomings of their predecessors were brought to the marketplace.[4,5,7,15] In the years between the 1990s and today, ankle replacement has gained popularity to the point that it is becoming the viable, accepted alternative for certain patients with end-stage ankle arthritis.[3–5,7,16–28]

ANKLE JOINT BIOMECHANICS

The nature and function of the ankle joint itself necessitated improved implant design from the start.[16,17] The biomechanics of the ankle joint is unique because of its topography, its load-bearing characteristics, and its surrounding soft tissue tethers. The talocrural and subtalar joints endure forces up to five times body weight during gait,

PMSI Orthopedics, Pottstown, PA, USA
E-mail address: overley@pmsiforlife.com

Clin Podiatr Med Surg 29 (2012) 547–570
http://dx.doi.org/10.1016/j.cpm.2012.07.003
0891-8422/12/$ – see front matter © 2012 Elsevier Inc. All rights reserved.

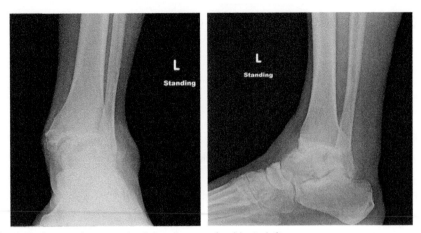

Fig. 1. End-stage degenerative joint disease of ankle. L, left.

which must be observed over a much smaller contact area than the hip and knee of the ipsilateral extremity. The smaller size of the joint leads to a higher resultant moment and higher compressive force.[16,17,29–31] The ankle joint also accepts two to three times the forces experienced by the hip or the knee, but only has one-third of the surface area to dissipate this load. Of greater concern is the available bone stock because the ankle joint has far less bone stock available for implantation of prosthetic replacement compared with the hip or the knee.[16,17,31]

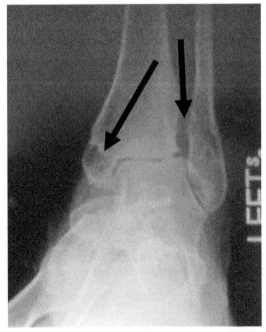

Fig. 2. Radiograph with healed medial malleolar and lateral malleolar fractures with an unaddressed syndesmotic injury and previous medial malleolar fracture (*see arrows*). Post-traumatic arthritic changes have occurred to the joint.

ARTHRODESIS VERSUS ARTHROPLASTY

There are many reports and studies by various investigators comparing ankle arthrodesis versus total ankle replacement. Haddad, SooHoo, Piriou, and Hintermann and their colleagues[32–36] all compared the satisfaction rates of the fused ankle versus ankle replacement versus healthy ankle joints themselves. The Barg and Hintermann[36] study showed that patients with fused ankles had 3% greater oxygen consumption than the ankle replacement group—yet another reason or impetus for developing an improved ankle replacement design. The study showed the stress on the additional joints when the ankle joint is fused and the impact of ankle fusion in significantly comorbid patient populations. The study also found the satisfaction rates of patients with replacements were 27% higher than patients who had ankle fusion. Piriou and colleagues[34] found that neither group (arthrodesis or arthroplasty) had normal movement restored. However, "the arthrodesis group had a faster gait; the arthroplasty group had a reduction of limping with gait." Piriou and colleagues[34] also found that the arthroplasty could demonstrate more of a symmetric gait and timing when compared with the arthrodesis group.

SURGICAL APPROACH

Ankle replacement requires the surgeon to incise the capsule to the periosteal layer and remove any osteophytes. The surgeon is required to use a combination of anterior or anterolateral surgical approaches for some of the older designs. Generally, the implant requires good exposure of the ankle joint. Exposure of the tubercle of Chaput is made to allow better visualization for insertion of the implant and to reduce stress on the soft tissues.

HISTORICAL OVERVIEW AND THE FIRST GENERATION OF ANKLE IMPLANTS

From a historical standpoint, there are three accepted generations of ankle replacement designs.[37–42] Despite this assessment, the categories on which these are based are market introduction to the general populace. Often, implants may straddle two or more generations. Examples include Scandinavian Total Ankle Replacement (STAR, Morrisville, PA, USA), TNK First Generation (Japan), and the Agility Ankle (DePuy, Warsaw, IN, USA).

In the early and middle 1970s reports appeared of early success with first generation implants in 80% to 85% of patients. In 11 reports that included 346 arthroplasties, good or fair results were reported in 83% and failures in 17%, at a mean follow-up of fewer than 5 years.[43–46]

Because of these promising results, the potential for total ankle arthroplasty as a viable surgical alternative peaked interest and the indications for the procedure were expanded to include patients who were younger with active lifestyles. Unfortunately, long-term follow-up reviews of early series of total ankle arthroplasties showed poor long-term results, especially in younger patients with isolated traumatic arthritis. In later reports, in which the average follow-up was longer than 5 years, failure occurred in 35% to 76% of arthroplasties.[8,43,47,48]

FIRST-GENERATION IMPLANTS

Marotte and Lord first implemented their reverse hip design for ankle replacement in the early 1970s (**Figs. 3–5**) with varied results in terms of satisfaction and success. Of the 25 implanted, only 7 were considered to be successful.[49] Consequently, the design was abandoned to the more predictable arthrodesis procedure. This initial design lost favor and new designs began to emerge. Designs such as the

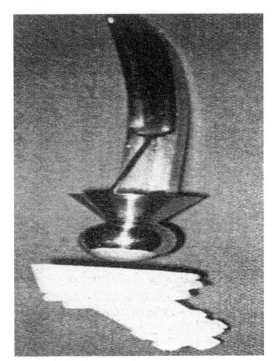

Fig. 3. Lord and Marotte "Total Ankle Replacement."

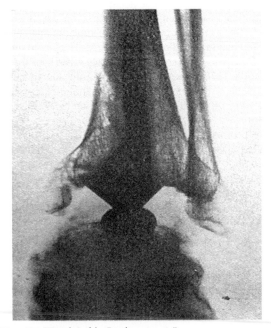

Fig. 4. Lord and Marotte "Total Ankle Replacement."

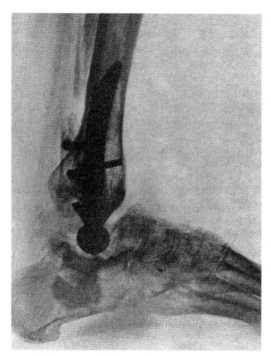

Fig. 5. Lord and Marotte "Total Ankle Replacement."

Mayo,[1,8,15] TNK First Generation,[50–58] and the first Buechel-Pappas Low Contact Stress[59,60] replacements were also received with skepticism during this same period. The MAYO success results were probably the most unsatisfactory of the first generation of ankle replacements between 1974 and 1984. Overall implant survival rate was 79% at 5 years, 65% at 10 years, and 61% at 15 years, with a revision rate of 41% for persistent pain according to Kitaoka and colleagues.[1] Unfortunately, total ankle replacement as a viable surgical procedure hit yet another stumbling block.

The reasons for the initial poor results from total ankle replacement included use of cemented designs; a unappreciated or lack of recognition of coronal malalignment; inferior metallurgy or implant composition; too much surgical "eyeballing," which led to overaggressive bone resection; and, finally, not fully understanding which cases were ideal for the procedure. These early mistakes led researchers and surgeons to refine implant design in hopes of increased success rates for total ankle replacement.[1,7] To overcome the negative stigma associated with early total ankle replacement, these designs had to show vast improvement over those that had failed during the 1970s. It was these early failures that set the stage for the second generation of implants. An overall industry and surgeon-related push was made to come up with designs that could reproduce near anatomic ankle motion. These designs had to be supportive and resist implant failure. New designs also required improved metallurgy for support.

Ankle Anatomy Relative to Implant Design Strategy

In terms of ankle anatomy and biomechanics, the improvement of ankle replacements had to address a few issues, including subsidence or loosening of the components on the talar or tibial side—the main reasons for implant failure.[16,17] Taking into account the overall long-term failures of the first generation of total ankle implants and a closer look at the structural shortcomings of the joint itself were instrumental in providing more robust and stable designs.

Tibial Component

In 1985, Hvid and colleagues[61] showed the greatest bone strength is in the postero-medial tibial plafond (**Fig. 6**) and the region of least bone strength is in the anterolateral tibia. Implant designs improved in their ability to disperse the weight load from the distal tibial plafond away from the weakest points and toward the stronger posterome-dial regions.[61] This forced transmission is eccentric and essentially loads on the cortical rim of the outside weightbearing surface as described by Trouillier and colleagues[62] in 2003 (**Fig. 7**). More current designs have addressed this issue in terms of their implantation or the stress applied across the implant surface from the distal tibia in hopes of preventing subsidence.[63,64]

Talar Component

The talar component implants have also evolved with new designs. Initial designs called for table-top cutting of the talus and nonisometric load and nonminimizing stress distribution. This practice led to subsidence and sinking of the talar components into the soft talar bone located just inside the anatomic talar wall perimeter. Newer designs have sought to maximize stress distribution while minimizing stress load by making more anatomic designs. The newer talar component designs not only disperse the vertical load to the outer rim of the talus where the stronger bone is found, but also prevent rotation that can lead to edge-loading and subsidence (**Fig. 8**).

SECOND-GENERATION IMPLANTS

The first second-generation total ankle replacements were designed or developed between 1979 and 2000. These include, but are no limited to, the first generation of STAR, the Agility Ankle (designed by Dr Frank Alvine; Food and Drug Administration [FDA] approval in 1995), and the Buechel-Pappas Low Contact Stress design (limited implantation) (**Fig. 9**).

In 2002, Easley and colleagues[22] stated that four second-generation total ankle arthroplasty designs showed reasonable functional outcomes: (1) STAR, (2) the Agility Ankle, (3) the Buechel-Pappas Total Ankle Replacement, and (4) the TNK ankle.

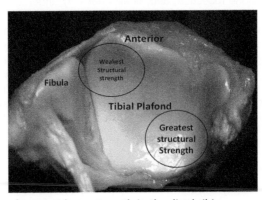

Fig. 6. The regions of greatest bone strength in the distal tibia.

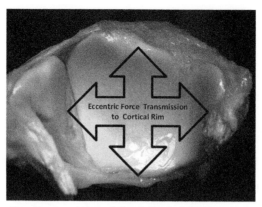

Fig. 7. Load distribution characteristics of distal tibial plafond.

Although the Agility Ankle is noted here, intermediate results are promising but should be treated with caution. In 2004, Knecht and colleagues[65–69] stated that arthrodesis of the tibiofibular syndesmosis impacts the radiographic and clinical outcomes with the Agility Ankle. The relatively low rates of radiographic hind-foot arthritis and revision procedures at an average of 9 years after the arthroplasty are encouraging. Replacement with the Agility Ankle was found to be a viable and durable option for the treatment of ankle arthritis in selected patients.[15,70–73]

The Agility Ankle can be classified as a fixed, semiconstrained implant because the polyethylene is fixed to the tibial tray (see **Fig. 8**). It is also considered a semiconstrained implant because it does not completely rely on soft tissue adaptability, although it does take it into account. The Agility Ankle uses external fixation to allow for exposure to the ankle joint during implantation. This design requires performing a distal fibular roll out on the lateral ankle joint side of the implant, as well as a synostosis of the distal tibia and fibula, which allows for appropriate component seating. The talar component is flanged to disperse vertical load force laterally to talar cortical rim, thereby decreasing the risk of subsidence. This talar modification has proved to be more successful then the previous nonflanged design of the early Agility Ankle (**Figs. 10** and **11**).

STAR (see **Fig. 11**, **Figs. 12–16**), designed by Dr Kofoed in 1979, has also undergone some redesigns and was introduced in the United States in 2010 (SBI, Small

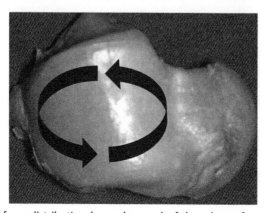

Fig. 8. Rotational force distribution (*curved arrows*) of the talar surface.

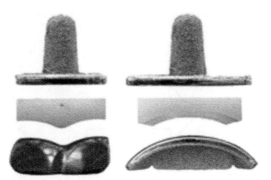

Fig. 9. Buechel-Pappas Low Contact Stress ankle implant.

Bone Innovations, Morrisville, PA, USA). The key features are its double-keeled distal tibial component, the sagittal design of the talar component, and its mobile bearing polyethylene design to decrease excessive contact and minimize stress fatigue. This also allows dynamic motion via the prosthesis by the mobility of the actual polyethylene meniscal component. The design has a radio opaque filament, which resides within the meniscal component. This design feature is helpful in demonstrating polyethylene fracture without operative determination.[74,75] Alignment is accomplished with a sagittal alignment guide that is pinned to the anterior tibia (see **Fig. 13**). This guide allows for accurate resection of the distal tibia as well as mediolateral and rotational translation to ensure appropriate postoperative alignment (see **Fig. 12**).

There have been six major revisions of the STAR implant since its inception in 1979, which shows the need for an organic improvement process for any successful design. The STAR is the only FDA-approved total ankle replacement system in the second generation that does not require cement.[31,67,74,76–83]

Other second-generation designs of note are the Ankle Evolution System,[74,84–86] the Mobility (DePuy), the Hintegra (Integra Life Sciences, Plainfield, NJ, USA) **(Figs. 17–19)**,

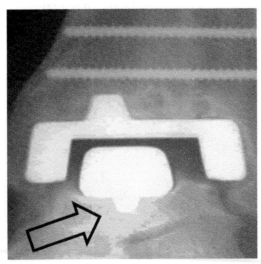

Fig. 10. Early design of Agility ankle implant with talar subsidence (*demonstrated by arrow*).

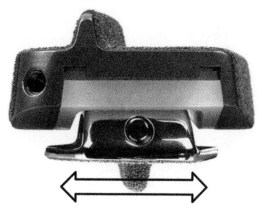

Fig. 11. New Agility total ankle replacement with "flanged" talar component (*represented by arrow*).

and other designs such as the TNK, which has been in use in Japan since the 1970s (**Fig. 20**).

THIRD-GENERATION IMPLANTS

The most recent generation of implants have similar characteristics to the second generation of total ankle replacement systems, however, there are a few marked and distinct differences of design with these implants.

Design Criteria

The design criteria used in total ankle replacement in some of the second and all of the third generations of implants can be sorted into five categories based on the nature of the joint and the implant interaction. These criteria are shown in **Fig. 21**.

The designs can be cemented or not cemented. Conformity characteristics are defined as the implant's ability to conform to the anatomy in which it is being implanted. Congrueny is defined as the implant's relationship to the other components of the implant and how they interact with multiplanar loading from the anatomy. Bearing types and constraint are directly interrelated in their ability to allow or disallow

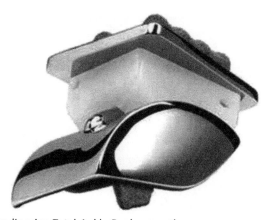

Fig. 12. STAR (Scandinavian Total Ankle Replacement).

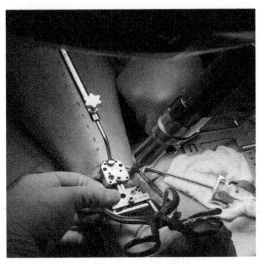

Fig. 13. Alignment guide for STAR total ankle replacement.

certain types of movement by restriction enforced either by the implant or by the anatomy. This concept is probably the most difficult to understand because it encompasses all aspects of the ankle itself, including ligament and/or tendon stability and strength in direct proportion to the allowable motion from the implant itself. This defined resistance of an implant to a particular degree of freedom in the anterior plane, posterior plane, or the axial rotation plane can be difficult to appreciate at first inspection. The early lack of attention to these criteria in the design of ankle replacement components may have contributed in part or solely to the early failures of these implants.[1]

The designs of note currently being used in the United States are the INBONE 1 and INBONE 2 (Wright Medical Technologies Brentwood, TN, USA) (**Figs. 22–24**), Salto Talaris (Tornier) (**Figs. 25–27**), STAR, and the updated, second-generation Agility Ankle.

The INBONE 1 and 2 designs use an extremity holder (**Fig. 28**) to secure the foot, ankle, and leg in appropriate alignment during the procedure. This holder allows the

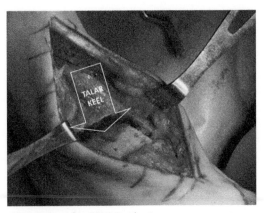

Fig. 14. Ankle joint preparation for STAR Implant.

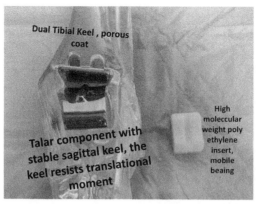

Fig. 15. STAR components.

surgeon to manipulate the extremity in multiple planes to ensure appropriate chamfer (guide) cutting and postoperative alignment. The tibial stemmed components can also provide support by bypassing cystic or soft areas of distal tibial metaphyseal bone for the denser bone in the diaphyseal-metaphyseal regions. The talar cut is a table-top cut, which is then affixed with a centrally stemmed talar component (INBONE 1; see **Figs. 22** and **24**) or a pillared talar component. The greatest disadvantages of this implant are the large bone resection required and the transtalar drilling approach to the ankle mortise.

The Salto Talaris has a fixed component, semiconstrained design. It features a single tibial keel, which resides in the stronger metaphyseal-diaphyseal juncture of the distal tibial. The single-keel design prevents rotation and anterior posterior migration. The talar component is unique in that it is essentially a talar resurfacing with only an anterior shaping with posterior and lateral cuts. These cuts, in theory, should eliminate any unwanted sacrifice of the deltoid arterial branch to the talar body and, thereby, reduce the chances of iatrogenic talar body bone necrosis. The alignment guide for the tibia is similar to that of the STAR implant, allowing for resectional depth of the tibia plafond to

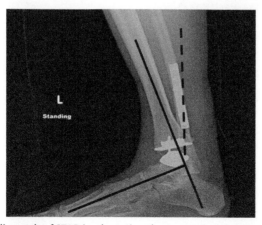

Fig. 16. Lateral radiograph of STAR implantation demonstrating postoperative dorsiflexion. L, left.

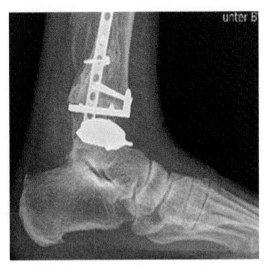

Fig. 17. Ankle Evolution System.

be adjusted, as well as adjusting for varus and valgus rotation and medial-lateral translation.

These designs share the ability to reduce vertical stress load across the ankle joint (a significant improvement) and the sulcus design or cleft of the talar components, which resist translational movement and also rotational movement of the implant

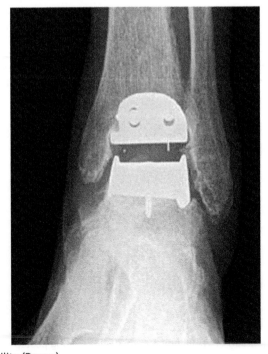

Fig. 18. The Mobility (Depuy).

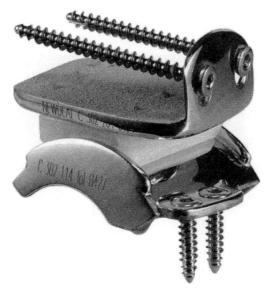

Fig. 19. Hintegra Total Ankle (Integra).

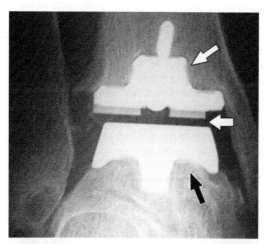

Fig. 20. TNK total ankle implant Tibial component (*superior white arrow*), Polyethylene insert (*middle white arrow*), Talar component (*inferior black arrow*).

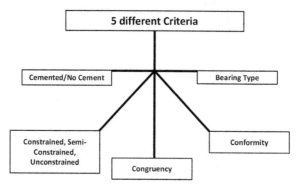

Fig. 21. Design criteria for total ankle replacements.

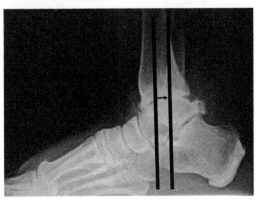

Fig. 22. Retrolisthesis or posterior displacement of the vertical mechanical axis of the talus relative to the vertical mechanical axis of the Tibia.

and the polyethylene component in an affixed or nonfixed mobile-bearing design. These new developments, coupled with new metallurgical porous coating linings for the tibial and talar components and high molecular weight polyethylene inserts, have the potential for increased survivorship and subsidence reduction (**Fig. 29**).

Over the last 3 to 4 years, the newer generation implant designs have led to improvement in overall satisfaction rates for the implants as well as in patient satisfaction. Indications for this type of procedure have broadened. With the improvement in overall surgical targeting and instrumentation, surgeons are more confident with total ankle replacements versus ankle arthrodesis. As a result, the numbers of total ankle replacements in the United States have significantly increased.[63,87–89] Over the last several years, the success rates of this procedure have improved significantly, thereby dispelling some of the earlier skepticism associated with total ankle replacement (**Fig. 30**).

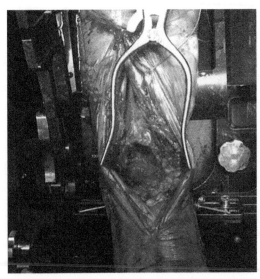

Fig. 23. Note the large amount of bone resection required for implantation.

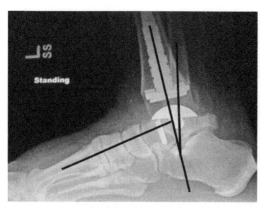

Fig. 24. Postoperative appearance after INBONE 1 Total Ankle Replacement with improvement in tibiotalar relationship and improved dorsiflexion. Lines represent increased Dorsiflexion of the Ankle Joint after ankle replacement.

Indications and Contraindications

Understanding the indications for implantation is of paramount importance to successful total ankle replacement. Indications have broadened since the advent of the second-generation and third-generation designs. These improvements provide a total ankle replacement option to a greater population of patients, leading to better satisfaction and improvement in overall quality of life.[26,90–97] This is a result of the improved surgical instrumentation and targeting designs and the improvement of surgeons' ability to select the appropriate cases.

Certainly, most patients with end-stage ankle arthritis can qualify for total ankle replacement. However, patients who are unstable diabetics or are suspected of

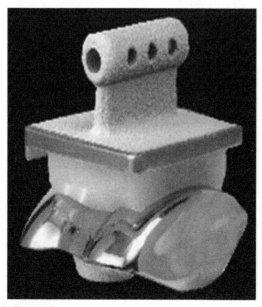

Fig. 25. Salto Talaris (Tornier).

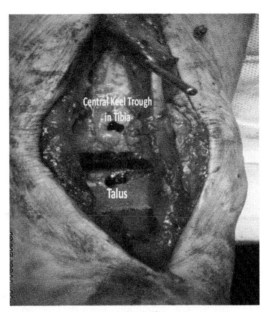

Fig. 26. Salto Talaris intraoperative appearance after osteotomy.

having a neuropathic ankle joint are excluded from total ankle replacement.[98] Less defined indications, such as gouty arthritis or avascular or aseptic necrosis of the talus or distal tibia, also have mixed results; however, these indication do not completely preclude ankle replacements.[98] Obviously, patients with insufficient bone stock in either the talar or distal tibial regions should be treated with extreme caution because this may result in subsidence even with sufficient grafting and in the best of hands.[99] Patients with any suspected circulatory deficit or infectious process (acute or chronic) should also be adequately evaluated before implantation and, if there is any concern, not be considered candidates for replacement.[98]

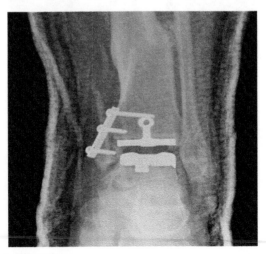

Fig. 27. Salto Talaris (Tornier).

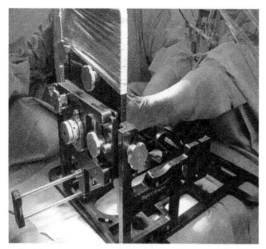

Fig. 28. INBONE Foot holder and targeting guide.

Alignment

In a 2003 review, Hintermann and Valderrabano[98] found that, although the results of the different design approaches are encouraging in limited clinical series, there is still the need for careful, long-term analyses to estimate to what extent the current designs are mimicking the biomechanics of the ankle joint. More attention must be paid to more accurate implantation techniques that result in well-balanced ligaments that act together with the replaced surfaces in a most physiologic manner. In 2004, Gill[29] noted that there is a need for further basic scientific research in total ankle arthroplasty. The lessons learned from other arthroplasties should be considered in ankle arthroplasty design. In 2004, Haskell and Mann[100] tested the hypotheses that

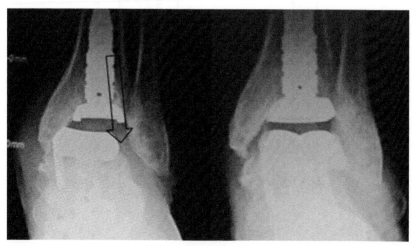

Fig. 29. Coronal malalignment of the ankle status after total ankle replacement and reimplantation with a cleft talar component. Note improvement of postoperative alignment and overall position. Arrow demonstrates "rotational (coronal) malalignment of the talar component and subsidence".

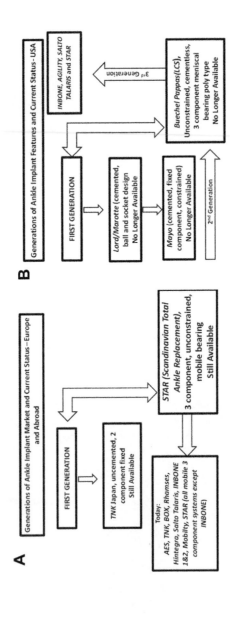

Fig. 30. (A) Europe and abroad first-generation total ankle implants. (B) United States first-generation and second-generation total ankle implants.

preoperative coronal plane malalignment and incongruence of the ankle can be corrected and maintained for 2 years with total ankle replacement. These investigators found that patients with preoperative incongruent joints are 10 times more likely to have progressive edge-loading develop than patients with congruent joints do. They state that surgeons must be attentive to coronal plane alignment during and after ankle replacement, and that longer follow-up is needed to assess the longevity of the correction and the impact of minor malalignment on implant wear.

SUMMARY

In short, although the implants themselves have improved, our ability to understand the way the ankle functions has also improved.[16,17,61] We still are learning and continue to learn with further developments in design and surgical technique. Consequently, our success rates should improve if we adhere to the following guidelines. Appropriate patient selection for total ankle replacement should be a priority. Other considerations include appropriate surgical technique, appreciation of soft tissue deficits present at the time of implantation, and appropriate staging of additional surgical procedures to correct coronal or sagittal malalignment issues. In addition, adhering to a strict and sound postoperative protocol will result in a greater likelihood of success for the patient and the implant.

Total ankle replacement surgery is on the rise mostly because of the new implantation techniques and design. As the designs continue to improve and the procedure is better refined, total ankle replacement should continue to be accepted at a greater level based on the mission statements of The American College of Foot and Ankle Surgeons and the American Orthopedic Foot and Ankle Society.[25]

ACKNOWLEDGMENTS

Special thanks and consideration to Michelle Sparks, DPM, PGY3 and Ashley Herczeg, DPM, PGY1 (Mercy Suburban Hospital, Norristown, Pa) who provided assistance in the editing and organization of this article.

REFERENCES

1. Conti SF, Wong YS. Complications of total ankle replacement. Clin Orthop 2001; 391:105–14.
2. Rockett MS, Ng A, Guimet M. Posttraumatic ankle arthrosis. Clin Podiatr Med Surg 2001;18(3):515–35.
3. Saltzman CL. Perspective on total ankle replacement. Foot Ankle Clin 2000;5(4): 761–75.
4. Gould JS, Alvine FG, Mann RA, et al. Total ankle replacement: a surgical discussion. Part II. The clinical and surgical experience. Am J Orthop 2000;29(9): 675–82.
5. Gould JS, Alvine FG, Mann RA, et al. Total ankle replacement: a surgical discussion. Part I. Replacement systems, indications, and contraindications. Am J Orthop 2000;29(8):604–9.
6. Cheng YM, Huang PJ, Hung SH, et al. The surgical treatment for degenerative disease of the ankle. Int Orthop 2000;24(1):36–9.
7. Saltzman CL, McIff TE, Buckwalter JA, et al. Total ankle replacement revisited. J Orthop Sports Phys Ther 2000;30(2):56–67.
8. Kitaoka HB, Patzer GL, Ilstrup DM, et al. Survivorship analysis of the Mayo total ankle arthroplasty. J Bone Joint Surg Am 1994;76(7):974–9.

9. Kitaoka HB. Fusion techniques for failed total ankle arthroplasty. Semin Arthroplasty 1992;3(1):51–7.
10. Kitaoka HB. Salvage of nonunion following ankle arthrodesis for failed total ankle arthroplasty. Clin Orthop 1991;268:37–43.
11. Alvine FG. Total ankle arthroplasty: new concepts and approaches. Contemp Orthop 1991;22(4):397–403.
12. Cuckler JM, Rhoad RC. Alternatives to hip, knee, and ankle total joint arthroplasty. Curr Opin Rheumatol 1991;3(1):81–7.
13. Dini AA, Bassett FH 3rd. Evaluation of the early result of Smith total ankle replacement. Clin Orthop 1980;146:228–30.
14. Kitaoka HB, Patzer GL. Clinical results of the Mayo total ankle arthroplasty. J Bone Joint Surg Am 1996;78(11):1658–64.
15. Pyevich MT, Saltzman CL, Callaghan JJ, et al. Total ankle arthroplasty: a unique design. Two to twelve-year follow-up. J Bone Joint Surg Am 1998;80(10):1410–20.
16. Deland JT, Morris GD, Sung IH. Biomechanics of the ankle joint. A perspective on total ankle replacement. Foot Ankle Clin 2000;5(4):747–59.
17. Neufeld SK, Lee TH. Total ankle arthroplasty: indications, results, and biomechanical rationale. Am J Orthop 2000;29(8):593–602.
18. Wood PL, Frcs MB, Clough TM, et al. Clinical comparison of two total ankle replacements. Foot Ankle Int 2000;21(7):546–50.
19. Saltzman CL. Total ankle arthroplasty: state of the art. Instr Course Lect 1999;48:263–8.
20. Lachiewicz PF. Rheumatoid arthritis of the ankle: the role of total ankle arthroplasty. Semin Arthroplasty 1995;6(3):187–92.
21. Lachiewicz PF. Total ankle arthroplasty. Indications, techniques, and results. Orthop Rev 1994;23(4):315–20.
22. Easley ME, Vertullo CJ, Urban WC, et al. Total ankle arthroplasty. J Am Acad Orthop Surg 2002;10(3):157–67.
23. Myerson MS, Miller SD. Salvage after complications of total ankle arthroplasty. Foot Ankle Clin 2002;7(1):191–206.
24. National Public Health Service for Wales. How effective are ankle replacement operations? What is the expected lifespan of a new ankle? ATTRACT Database. Gwent (Wales): National Public Health Service for Wales; 2001. Available at: http://www.attract.wales.nhs.uk/question_answers.cfm?question_id=208. Accessed September 30, 2005.
25. American Orthopaedic Foot and Ankle Society (AOFAS). AOFAS position statement: total ankle arthroplasty. Seattle (WA): AOFAS; 2003. Available at: http://www.aofas.org/displaycommon.cfm?an=1&subarticlenbr=27. Accessed September 21, 2005.
26. Valderrabano V, Pagenstert G, Horisberger M, et al. Sports and recreation activity of ankle arthritis patients before and after total ankle replacement. Am J Sports Med 2006;34(6):993–9.
27. Bonasia DE, Dettoni F, Femino JE, et al. Total ankle replacement: why, when and how? Iowa Orthop J 2010;30:119–30.
28. Park JS, Mroczek KJ. Total ankle arthroplasty. Bull NYU Hosp Jt Dis 2011;69(1):27–35.
29. Gill LH. Challenges in total ankle arthroplasty. Foot Ankle Int 2004;25(4):195–207.
30. Spirt AA, Assal M, Hansen ST Jr. Complications and failure after total ankle arthroplasty. J Bone Joint Surg Am 2004;86-A(6):1172–8.

31. Benedetti MG, Leardini A, Romagnoli M, et al. Functional outcome of meniscal-bearing total ankle replacement: a gait analysis study. J Am Podiatr Med Assoc 2008;98(1):19–26.
32. Haddad SL, Coetzee JC, Estok R, et al. Intermediate and long-term outcomes of total ankle arthroplasty and ankle arthrodesis. A systematic review of the literature. J Bone Joint Surg Am 2007;89(9):1899–905.
33. SooHoo NF, Zingmond DS, Ko CY. Comparison of reoperation rates following ankle arthrodesis and total ankle arthroplasty. J Bone Joint Surg Am 2007; 89(10):2143–9.
34. Piriou P, Culpan P, Mullins M, et al. Ankle replacement versus arthrodesis: a comparative gait analysis study. Foot Ankle Int 2008;29(1):3–9.
35. Wood PL, Sutton C, Mishra V, et al. A randomised, controlled trial of two mobile-bearing total ankle replacements. J Bone Joint Surg Br 2009;91(1):69–74.
36. Barg A, Hintermann B. Take down of painful fusion and conversion into total ankle arthroplasty. J Am Acad Orthop Surg 2008;850–8.
37. Vickerstaff JA, Miles AW, Cunningham JL. A brief history of total ankle replacement and a review of the current status. Med Eng Phys 2007;29(10):1056–64.
38. Yalamanchili P, Neufeld S, Lin S. Total ankle arthroplasty: a modern perspective. Curr Orthop Prac 2009;20(2):106–10.
39. Slobogean GP, Younger A, Apostle KL, et al. Preference-based quality of life of end-stage ankle arthritis treated with arthroplasty or arthrodesis. Foot Ankle Int 2010;31(7):563–6.
40. Small Bone Innovations Inc. (SBi). Designed specifically for the small bone and joint surgeon: S.T.A.R. Ankle implants and instruments guide. MKT 16011 Rev. E 03/10. Morrisville (PA): SBi; 2010.
41. Raikin SM. Total ankle arthroplasty. Orthopedics 2010;33(12):890–1.
42. DiDomenico LA, Treadwell JR, Cain LZ. Total ankle arthroplasty in the rheumatoid patient. Clin Podiatr Med Surg 2010;27(2):295–311.
43. Helm R, Stevens J. Long-term results of total ankle replacement. J Arthroplasty 1986;1(4):271–7.
44. Lachiewicz PF, Inglis AE, Ranawat CS. Total ankle replacement in rheumatoid arthritis. J Bone Joint Surg Am 1984;66(3):340–3.
45. Kaukonen JP, Raunio P. Total ankle replacement in rheumatoid arthritis: a preliminary review of 28 arthroplasties in 24 patients. Ann Chir Gynaecol 1983;72(4): 196–9.
46. Smith CL. Physical therapy management of patients with total ankle replacement. Phys Ther 1980;60(3):303–6.
47. Kitaoka HB, Romness DW. Arthrodesis for failed ankle arthroplasty. J Arthroplasty 1992;7(3):277–84.
48. Wynn AH, Wilde AH. Long-term follow-up of the Conaxial (Beck-Steffee) total ankle arthroplasty. Foot Ankle 1992;13(6):303–6.
49. Guyton JR. Arthroplasty of the hip and knee. In: Canale ST, editor. Campbell's operative orthopedics, vol. 6, 9th edition. St Louis (MO): C.V. Mosby Inc; 1998. p. 232–5.
50. Takakura Y, Tanaka Y, Sugimoto K, et al. Ankle arthroplasty. A comparative study of cemented metal and uncemented ceramic prostheses. Clin Orthop 1990;252: 209–16.
51. Das AK Jr. Total ankle arthroplasty: a review of 37 cases. J Tenn Med Assoc 1988;81(11):682–5.
52. Spaulding JM, Megesi RG, Figgie HE 3rd, et al. Total ankle arthroplasty. A procedural review. AORN J 1988;48(2):201–3, 206–7, 210–2 passim.

53. Unger AS, Inglis AE, Mow CS, et al. Total ankle arthroplasty in rheumatoid arthritis: a long-term follow-up study. Foot Ankle 1988;8(4):173–9.
54. Scholz KC. Total ankle arthroplasty using biological fixation components compared to ankle arthrodesis. Orthopedics 1987;10(1):125–31.
55. Bolton-Maggs BG, Sudlow RA, Freeman MA. Total ankle arthroplasty. A long-term review of the London Hospital experience. J Bone Joint Surg Br 1985; 67(5):785–90.
56. Stauffer RN. Salvage of painful total ankle arthroplasty. Clin Orthop 1982;170: 184–8.
57. Demottaz JD, Mazur JM, Thomas WH, et al. Clinical study of total ankle replacement with gait analysis. A preliminary report. J Bone Joint Surg Am 1979;61(7): 976–88.
58. Nizard R. Computer assisted surgery for total knee arthroplasty. Acta Orthop Belg 2002;68(3):215–30.
59. Buechel FF, Pappas MJ. Survivorship and clinical evaluation of cementless, meniscal-bearing total ankle replacements. Semin Arthroplasty 1992;3(1): 43–50.
60. Buechel FF, Pappas MJ, Iorio LJ. New Jersey low contact stress total ankle replacement: biomechanical rationale and review of 23 cementless cases. Foot Ankle 1988;8(6):279–90.
61. Hvid I, Rasmussen O, Jensen NC, et al. Trabecular bone strength profiles at the ankle joint. Clin Orthop Relat Res 1985;199:306–12.
62. Trouillier H, Hänsel L, Schaff P, et al. Long-term results after ankle arthrodesis: clinical, radiological, gait analytical aspects. Foot Ankle Int 2002;23(12): 1081–90.
63. Deorio JK, Easley ME. Total ankle arthroplasty. Instr Course Lect 2008;57: 383–413.
64. Chou LB, Coughlin MT, Hansen S Jr, et al. Osteoarthritis of the ankle: the role of arthroplasty. J Am Acad Orthop Surg 2008;16(5):249–59.
65. Knecht SI, Estin M, Callaghan JJ, et al. The Agility total ankle arthroplasty. Seven to sixteen-year follow-up. J Bone Joint Surg Am 2004;86-A(6):1161–71.
66. McGarvey WC, Clanton TO, Lunz D. Malleolar fracture after total ankle arthroplasty: a comparison of two designs. Clin Orthop Relat Res 2004;424: 104–10.
67. Anderson T, Montgomery F, Carlsson A. Uncemented STAR total ankle prostheses. J Bone Joint Surg Am 2004;86-A(Suppl 1(Pt 2)):103–11.
68. Tarasevicius S, Tarasevicius R, Kalesinskas RJ, et al. Early results of total ankle arthroplasty. Medicina (Kaunas) 2004;40(4):327–31 [in Lithuanian].
69. Stengel D, Bauwens K, Ekkernkamp A, et al. Efficacy of total ankle replacement with meniscal-bearing devices: a systematic review and meta-analysis. Arch Orthop Trauma Surg 2005;125(2):109–19.
70. Schuberth JM, Patel S, Zarutsky E. Perioperative complications of the Agility total ankle replacement in 50 initial, consecutive cases. J Foot Ankle Surg 2006;45(3):139–46.
71. Kopp FJ, Patel MM, Deland JT, et al. Total ankle arthroplasty with the Agility prosthesis: clinical and radiographic evaluation. Foot Ankle Int 2006;27(2):97–103.
72. Raikin SM, Myerson MS. Avoiding and managing complications of the Agility Total Ankle Replacement system. Orthopedics 2006;29(10):930–8.
73. Van der Heide HJ, Novakova I, de Waal Malefijt MC. The feasibility of total ankle prosthesis for severe arthropathy in haemophilia and prothrombin deficiency. Haemophilia 2006;12(6):679–82.

74. Kharwadkar N, Harris NJ. Revision of STAR total ankle replacement to hybrid AES-STAR total ankle replacement—a report of two cases. Foot Ankle Surg 2009;15(2):101–5.
75. Scott AT, Nunley JA. Polyethylene fracture following STAR ankle arthroplasty: a report of three cases. Foot Ankle Int 2009;30(4):375–9.
76. Murnaghan JM, Warnock DS, Henderson SA. Total ankle replacement. Early experiences with STAR prosthesis. Ulster Med J 2005;74(1):9–13.
77. Carlsson A, Markusson P, Sundberg M. Radiostereometric analysis of the double-coated STAR total ankle prosthesis: a 3–5 year follow-up of 5 cases with rheumatoid arthritis and 5 cases with osteoarthrosis. Acta Orthop 2005; 76(4):573–9.
78. Henricson A, Skoog A, Carlsson A. The Swedish Ankle Arthroplasty Register: an analysis of 531 arthroplasties between 1993 and 2005. Acta Orthop 2007;78(5): 569–74.
79. Martin RL, Stewart GW, Conti SF. Posttraumatic ankle arthritis: an update on conservative and surgical management. J Orthop Sports Phys Ther 2007; 37(5):253–9.
80. Cracchiolo A, DeOrio JK. Design features of current total ankle replacements: implants and instrumentation. J Am Acad Orthop Surg 2008;16:530–40.
81. Wood PL, Prem H, Sutton C. Total ankle replacement: medium-term results in 200 Scandinavian total ankle replacements. J Bone Joint Surg Br 2008;90(5): 605–9.
82. Saltzman CL, Mann RA, Ahrens JE, et al. Prospective controlled trial of STAR total ankle replacement versus ankle fusion: initial results. Foot Ankle Int 2009; 30(7):579–96.
83. Schutte BG, Louwerens JW. Short-term results of our first 49 Scandanavian total ankle replacements (STAR). Foot Ankle Int 2008;29(2):124–7.
84. Popelka S, Vavrík P, Landor I, et al. Our experience with AES total ankle replacement. Acta Chir Orthop Traumatol Cech 2010;77(1):24–31.
85. Morgan SS, Brooke B, Harris NJ. Total ankle replacement by the Ankle Evolution System: medium-term outcome. J Bone Joint Surg Br 2010;92(1):61–5.
86. Besse JL, Colombier JA, Asencio J, et al, l'AFCP. Total ankle arthroplasty in France. Orthop Traumatol Surg Res 2010;96(3):291–303.
87. Guyer AJ, Richardson G. Current concepts review: total ankle arthroplasty. Foot Ankle Int 2008;29(2):256–64.
88. Karantana A, Hobson S, Dhar S. The Scandinavian total ankle replacement: survivorship at 5 and 8 years comparable to other series. Clin Orthop Relat Res 2010;468(4):951–7.
89. Gougoulias N, Khanna A, Maffulli N. How successful are current ankle replacements?: a systematic review of the literature. Clin Orthop Relat Res 2010;468(1): 199–208.
90. Cimon K, Cunningham J. Total ankle replacements: clinical effectiveness and a review of the guidelines. Health Technology Inquiry Service (HTIS). Ottawa (Ontario): Canadian Agency for Drugs and Technologies in Health (CADTH); 2008.
91. Naal FD, Impellizzeri FM, Loibl M, et al. Habitual physical activity and sports participation after total ankle arthroplasty. Am J Sports Med 2009;37(1): 95–102.
92. Kofoed H, Lundberg-Jensen A. Ankle arthroplasty in patients younger and older than 50 years: a prospective series with long-term follow-up. Foot Ankle Int 1999;20(8):501–6.

93. Buechel FF Sr, Buechel FF Jr, Pappas MJ. Ten-year evaluation of cementless Buechel-Pappas meniscal bearing total ankle replacement. Foot Ankle Int 2003;24(6):462–72.

94. Hosman AH, Mason RB, Hobbs T, et al. A New Zealand national joint registry review of 202 total ankle replacements followed for up to 6 years. Acta Orthop 2007;78(5):584–91.

95. Bonnin MP, Laurent JR, Casillas M. Ankle function and sports activity after total ankle arthroplasty. Foot Ankle Int 2009;30(10):933–44.

96. Naal FD, Impellizzeri FM, Rippstein PF. Which are the most frequently used outcome instruments in studies on total ankle arthroplasty? Clin Orthop Relat Res 2010;468(3):815–26.

97. van den Heuvel A, Van Bouwel S, Dereymaeker G. Total ankle replacement. Design evolution and results. Acta Orthop Belg 2010;76(2):150–61.

98. Hintermann B, Valderrabano V. Total ankle replacement. Foot Ankle Clin 2003; 8(2):375–405.

99. Koivu H, Kohonen I, Sipola E, et al. Severe periprosthetic osteolytic lesions after the Ankle Evolutive System total ankle replacement. J Bone Joint Surg Br 2009; 91(7):907–14.

100. Haskell A, Mann RA. Ankle arthroplasty with preoperative coronal plane deformity: short-term results. Clin Orthop 2004;424:98–103.

Revision of Failed Ankle Implants

Lawrence A. DiDomenico, DPM[a,b,]*, Davina Cross, DPM[c]

KEYWORDS

- Total ankle joint replacement • Ankle joint arthrodesis • Degeneration • Arthritis

KEY POINTS

- TAR offers the benefit of perseveration of joint motion, with potential decreased occurrence of adjacent joint degeneration, and a more expedient path to weight bearing.
- Studies have demonstrated that the new generation of TAR systems provides superior patient satisfaction outcomes compared with prior systems and with ankle arthrodesis.
- A plantargrade foot type provides the optimal setting for application of TAR, and adjunctive procedures may be necessary to rectify concomitant biomechanical factors.

INTRODUCTION

Total ankle joint replacement (TAR) has been offered as an alternative to ankle joint arthrodesis since the 1970s. Historically, ankle arthrodesis has been viewed as the gold standard of treatment of end-stage arthritis, because it offers reliable reduction of pain with good functional outcomes.[1] However, as with any surgical endeavor there are complications, including nonunion, malalignment, and gait alterations. These issues, in addition to a tenuous postoperative course, may decrease patient satisfaction and functional outcomes. In addition, degeneration of joints adjacent to the ankle, specifically the subtalar joint, is a concern and may predispose the joints to arthritis after ankle arthrodesis has been performed.[2]

Alternately, TAR offers the benefit of perseveration of joint motion, with potential decreased occurrence of adjacent joint degeneration, and a more expedient path to weight bearing. Studies have demonstrated inherently better patient outcomes with ankle arthroplasties, when performed with the second-generation implants.[2,3]

Since their introduction, TAR devices have undergone a variety of modifications, specifically in regards to the number and type of components used. These modifications have been necessary because previous success rates of TAR long-term outcomes did not equivocate with those of total knee and hip replacements.[4,5] The reasoning behind this trend is thought to be multifactorial. It may be because a high proportion of patients suffering from degeneration of the ankle joint are often younger, more active

[a] Department of Podiatry, Department of Surgery, St. Elizabeth Health Center, Youngstown, Ohio, USA; [b] The Ankle and Foot Care Centers, Youngstown, Ohio 44512, USA; [c] Resident, Heritage Valley Health Systems, Beaver, PA, USA
* Corresponding author.
E-mail address: ld5353@aol.com

Clin Podiatr Med Surg 29 (2012) 571–584
http://dx.doi.org/10.1016/j.cpm.2012.08.001
0891-8422/12/$ – see front matter © 2012 Elsevier Inc. All rights reserved.

patients who have likely suffered a traumatic injury.[6] Generally, lower patient outcome scores have been related to younger populations, whereas higher rated outcomes are seen with older patients who have a smaller body mass index.[7]

OVERVIEW OF TAR AND SYSTEMS

Indications for TAR include posttraumatic osteoarthritis, systemic arthritis, primary arthritis, or revision from prior ankle arthrodesis.[3]

The early implant models were cemented, and constructed of two components, which were described as constrained, semiconstrained, or nonconstrained.[8] These early models proved to be unstable when applied, leading to high rates of failure and disappointing long-term results.[9,10]

The initial models were followed by a generation of three-component models that had a central component that allowed multiaxial motion of the joint.[8] The models used currently are typically cementless, with a mobile-bearing polyethylene component. Each of the available models varies in structure and composition. The Salto (Tornier SA, St. Ismier, France) device is composed of cobalt-chrome alloy, followed by a layer of pure titanium and calcium hydroxyapatite.[11] This hydroxyapatite layer is intended to decrease the occurrence of radiolucency surrounding the implant. Another commonly used implant device is the Agility Total Ankle System (DePuy, Warsaw, IN).[3] This product has two components, which are composed of titanium and cobalt-chromium, and is semiconstrained. Bone ingrowth is a key factor for secure implantation of this device because cement is not used for application.[3] In addition, this implant partially relies on fusion of the distal tibiofibular syndesmosis for added stability.[12]

The Scandinavian Total Ankle Replacement (STAR) has three uncemented components, and is considered to be a mobile-bearing unit. The tibial and talar components are composed of cobalt-chrome, with a double coat of titanium and calcium phosphate. The third piece is ultra-high molecular weight polyethylene.[9]

Another implant device is the AES (Ankle Evolution System, Biomet, Nimes, France). This is an uncemented, three-component, meniscal-bearing unit, offering a triangular-shaped tibial stem, which offers increased stability.[13]

Preoperative planning to prevent failure of TAR is a key component for positive outcomes. Chances for postoperative lack of range of motion, implant instability, and lack of fusion of the tibiofibular syndesmosis may be avoided with thorough preoperative evaluation of the mechanical axis of the causing deformity.[12] Furthermore, realistic expectations regarding outcomes after the procedure must be conveyed to the patient. Specifically, a decrease in the amount of ankle joint range of motion as compared with a normal joint is likely to be expected and has been documented.[14]

MECHANISMS OF FAILURE

Complications leading to failure of TAR can be caused by several factors. The necessity for revision may be linked to the type of implant system used, surgeon experience in performing the procedure, or the severity of the patient's preoperative condition. Specifically, it has been found that surgeon experience can be related to long-term survival rate of ankle implants. Research has shown that after the surgeon has performed the application of 30 implants, the 5-year success rate increases from 70% to 86% (**Fig. 1**).[11]

Historically, aseptic prosthetic loosening and wound healing issues were among the most common complications arising after TAR with mechanical loosening occurring most commonly.[2,8,11] Other problems that frequently occur include infection of bone

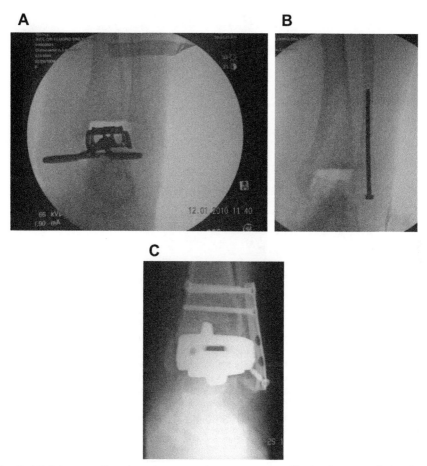

Fig. 1. (*A*) Intraoperative view demonstrating a transverse fibular fracture of the distal fibula. (*B*) Intraoperatively a 4.0 interfragmentary screw is used with a washer for compression and realignment of the distal fibular fracture. (*C*) Postoperative view demonstrating a medial malleolus fracture secondary to stress, and the medial malleolus was cut too thin.

and soft tissue, nonunion of the tibiofibular syndesmosis, malalignment, joint impingement, and persistent pain (**Fig. 2**).[5]

A thorough understanding of ankle joint anatomy is key for interpreting the mechanical and functional relationship between the prosthesis and joint, and may lend insight into mechanisms of failure.[15] Because of the lack of muscular reinforcement between the talus and surrounding bony structures, there is increased importance placed on the quality and integrity of the surrounding ligamentous structures (**Fig. 3**).[16]

One of the factors that make successful application of TAR inherently challenging is that many of the conditions that warrant the initial need for augmentation of the joint may cause complications after application. Preoperative failure to recognize inherent soft tissue or bony structural deformities contributes to this problem. Furthermore, inadequate soft tissue repair or component placement could be contributory factors to subsequent failure.[7,17] Tibiotalar varus or valgus have been linked to the highest incidence of complications.[6] It has been recommend that

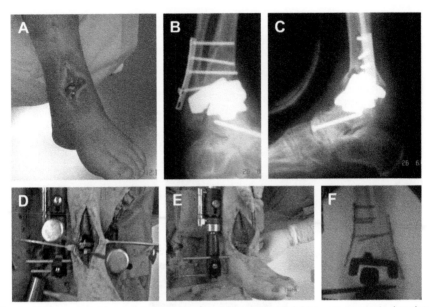

Fig. 2. (*A*) Rheumatoid patient postoperative with a wound dehissence. In particular, rheumatoid patients have a higher rate of wound complications because of the thin soft tissue envelope. (*B*) A patient who sustained a traumatic accident with a distal tibial fracture and subsidence of an Agility implant. (*C*) Lateral postoperative view after a traumatic accident with a distal tibial fracture and subsidence. (*D*) Intraoperative view demonstrating the amount of distal tibial bone loss from the subsidence. A trial implant is viewed demonstrating the amount of bone graft needed to secure the implant. (*E*) Intraoperative view demonstrating bone graft packed tightly into the distal tibia for the revision surgery. (*F*) Intraoperative view demonstrating the bone graft and the revision components of the Agility implant secured by a medial and lateral plate.

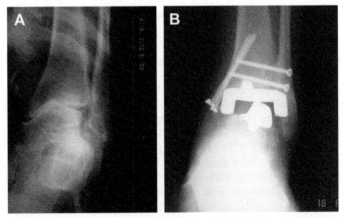

Fig. 3. (*A*) A patient with a varus ankle and ankle instability with loss of lateral ligamentous structures. (*B*) Postoperative view of a patient who had inadequate soft tissue repair and component placement, which led to this varus deformity and failure of the implant.

TAR procedures be avoided in patients with a coronal deformity of greater than 10 to 15 degrees.[18] In addition, equinus deformity has been noted to be an impacting factor in TAR, and some authors have recommended performing lengthening of the Achilles tendon if less than 5 degrees of dorsiflexion is achieved after placement of the implant.[11] This and other adjunctive procedures including osteotomies, arthrodesis, or tendon transfers may be necessary to provide the best environment for successful TAR outcomes (**Fig. 4**).

The type of implant used can be related to the mechanism of failure, depending on the shape, thickness, or angulation of the components. For example, osteolytic cysts have been demonstrated to develop more frequently in the uncemented, mobile-bearing implants. Wear debris particles or cysts are another sequalae that are thought to be caused by an unevenly loaded polyethylene component.[19] These cysts tend to weaken the stability of the implant, and may lead to implant loosening or fractures in the surrounding bone.[20]

Several indications for reoperation after TAR have been described. These include uncontrolled pain, along with radiographic evidence of component loosening, malpositioning, hypertrophic bone growth at the level of the implant, or signs of nonunion (**Fig. 5**).[3]

It is highly recommended that the surgeon acquire a CT scan before performing the revisional procedure to evaluate the surrounding bone stock.[20,21]

REVISIONAL RATES

Henricson and Agren[22] in a study examining 186 patients who had undergone previous TAR determined that the type of deformity present before the initial TAR may indicate the likelihood of the necessity of revisional surgery. In their research they found that revision rates for patients with a varus type of deformity was 31%, compared with 17% in those with either neutral or valgus position. The authors found an overall revision rate of 21%. Wood and Deakin[23] experienced 14 failures

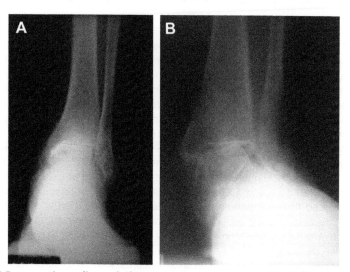

Fig. 4. (*A*) Preoperative radiograph demonstrating a congruent varus ankle. The axis of the tibial falls lateral to the central talus. (*B*) Preoperative radiograph clearly showing an incongruent ankle valgus secondary to medial deltoid insufficiency.

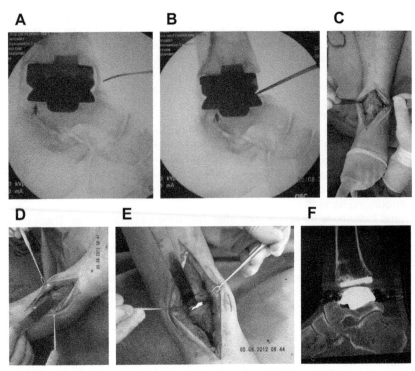

Fig. 5. (A) Intraoperative view demonstrating a large bony bridge over the anterior aspect of the implant, which limited the range of motion of the ankle joint. (B) Intraoperative lateral view after an aggressive resection of the hyptertrophic bone. (C–E) Intraoperative views demonstrating the hypertrophic bone (C), resecting of the hypertrophic bone with an osteotome (D), and after complete resection of hypertrophic bone anteriorly. (F) Preoperative CT scan displaying subsidence of the talar component of an Agility ankle replacement.

out of 200 patients who had had the STAR prosthesis in place. Zhao and colleagues[24] in a large systematic review of STAR failure rates in 2088 implants at mean follow-up of 52 months found 232 to be failed, for a combined failure rate of 11.1%. They found 11 primary complications, with the three earliest including loosening, deep infection, and malalignment. Additionally, Karantana and coworkers[9] reviewing 45 patients with STAR implants related that eight patients required revisional surgery consisting of component replacement (six) and arthrodesis (two).

Spirit and coworkers[3] in a review of 306 TAR procedures demonstrated the need for revisions in 86 patients. Of those requiring revision, 57 had one revision done at a mean of 17.8 months. Eighteen of the patients required two reoperations, and those were performed at 13.7 and 10.6 months post initial TAR, respectively. Nine of the patients required three reoperations, and those were performed at 10.8, 7.2, and 5 months, respectively. Lastly, one of the patients required seven reoperations.

Henricson and coworkers[13] in a review of 93 patients who had the AES ankle arthroplasties demonstrated a 5-year survival rate of 90%. Interestingly, the authors also reported a low revisional rate in their patients with rheumatoid arthritis (RA), which is beneficial because patients with systemic arthritidies often have poor bone quality.

REVISIONAL PROCEDURES AND METHODS

Henricson and coworkers[13] proposed the application of definitions to follow-up procedures for TAR. These included "revision," which entailed replacement or removal of the components, not including the polyethylene piece. "Reoperation" was another type, and this described surgery involving the joint but not the components. Finally, "additional procedure" was the term used for a secondary surgery not involving the ankle joint or the components. The type of reoperation procedure varies depending on the pathology present at or near the implant. Bony debridement, exchange of components, infection control, fracture or nonunion repair, extra-articular soft tissue procedures, and below-knee amputation have all been described.[3,13]

Redo-revision, or reapplication of an implant, has been found to be more difficult than revision converted to arthrodesis, primarily because of poor bone quality and availability, which is necessary to place a new implant.[2] In cases where this is the circumstance, or if there is surrounding soft tissue compromise, ankle arthrodesis may be the most viable revisional option.[5] The surgical technique for performing this procedure varies. Berkowitz and colleagues[5] detailed arthrodesis techniques in 24 patients who had previously undergone TAR. The incisional approach was similar to the original TAR, and the implant was removed using Arbeitsgemeinschaft für Osteosynthesefragen (AO) osteotomes. The authors further recommended thorough debridement of any excess synovial tissue in addition to acquisition of bone biopsy samples to rule out any infectious process.

Some surgeons have demonstrated the use of a retrograde intramedullary nail for revisional procedures.[25] Arthrodesis as a salvage procedure for previous TAR has been shown to have a reliable fusion rate, but this decreases in patients with RA.[26] Doets and Zurcher[26] in their review of 18 patients undergoing this procedure experienced seven nonunions, and all were in patients with inflammatory joint disease. Also in this study, the authors preferred fixation of the fusion site with either a blade plate for normative subtalar joints, or intramedullary-locking nails for degenerated joints. To promote fusion rates, use of structural bone graft to augment the arthrodesis site has also been highly recommended by several authors.[5,9,26] The use of the intramedullary nail in combination with a cage filled with morsellized cancellous bone grafting material has also been described.[27] This method offers stability with the cage apparatus, in combination with the superior biologic properties of the cancellous graft. However, alternately, there have been some reported failures of fusion when using this technique (**Fig. 6**).[28]

In instances where adequate bone stock remains and there is little soft tissue compromise, several authors have detailed success when removing the failing TAR device, and replacing it with a different style. Use of the Agility custom prosthesis has been recommended because of its customizable polyethylene thickness, stem angulation, diameter, and length.[20] This is accomplished by using preoperative radiographic templates to determine the appropriate sizing modifications. In addition, the tibial component can remain in place if it is in the proper position, and a specialized mismatch-type polyethylene piece can be used to approximate the two components.[20] Others have performed TAR conversion, creating a combination or hybrid system using STAR and AES components simultaneously. Specifically, Kharwadkar and Harris[29] presented two cases with excellent outcomes that entailed replacing only the STAR tibial components with the AES components, while preserving the STAR talar and polyethylene pieces (**Figs. 7** and **8**).

Bony overgrowth is a fairly common problem with TAR. This occurs secondary to subsidence of the talar component, and although a short-term solution may include

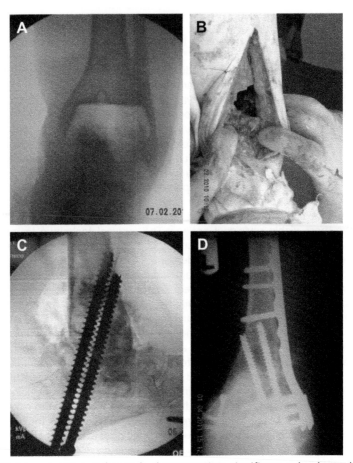

Fig. 6. (*A*) Intraoperative radiograph demonstrating significant talar bone loss after a trauma to an Agility ankle replacement several years postoperatively. Note the amount of bone void secondary to the trauma. (*B*) Intraoperative view after removal of the Agility implant demonstrating a large bone void after removal of the implant and the sustained bone loss. (*C*) Lateral intraoperative view with an autogenous cortical cancellous bone graft at the tibial calcaneal joint fixated with two fully threaded cancellous positional screws. (*D*) Postoperative view demonstrating complete incorporation of the autogenous bone graft, which is fixated with two large fully threaded cancellous positional screws and a femoral locking plate.

debridement within the medial and lateral gutters, it has been proposed that a more definitive method may include talar component revision, with application of a piece that covers more surface area (**Fig. 9**).[30]

Severe subsidence of the talar component can also cause tremendous bone loss. In these instances, it has been demonstrated that moderately successful revision can be achieved using an inbone-style implant.[31] Alternately, other authors have proposed using metal-reinforced cement augmentation, which has been previously used with success in other joint replacement revisions.[32] Another modification that has been used in patients with RA is augmentation of the tibia with hydroxyapatite.[33] However, in their review of TAR in 16 ankles in patients with RA, Shi and colleagues[33]

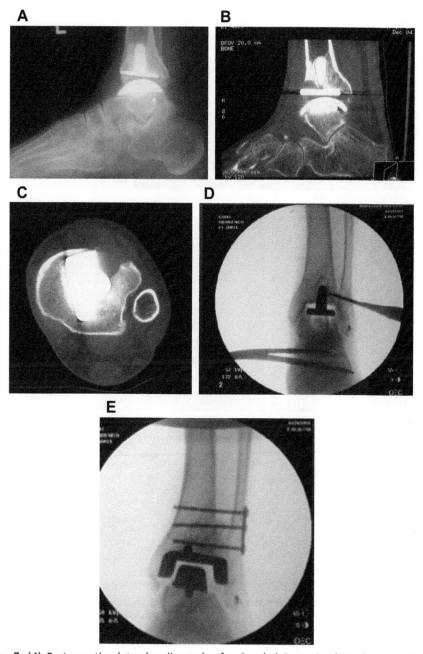

Fig. 7. (*A*) Postoperative lateral radiograph of a Buechel Papas implant demonstrating a distal tibial cyst and loosening of the tibial tray. (*B, C*) CT scans demonstrating the distal tibial cyst and the bone loss allowing for micromotion of the tibial tray of the Buechal Pappas implant. (*D*) Intraoperative view removing the tibial tray of the Buechal Pappas implant. (*E*) Intraoperative view demonstration of bone grafting of the bone void and insertion of an Agility implant.

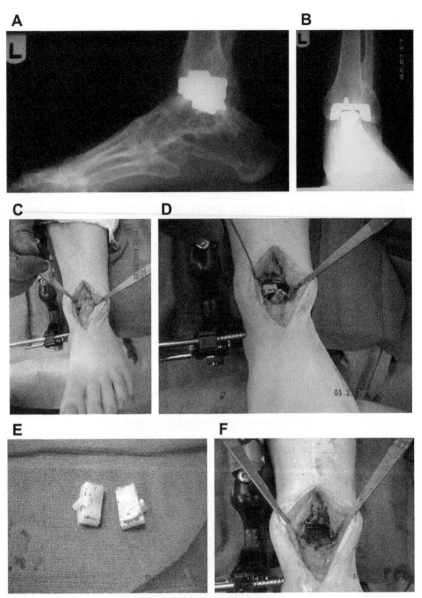

Fig. 8. (*A, B*) Preoperative anterolateral and lateral radiograph of a patient who had an Agility ankle replacement implanted approximately 12 years ago. The patient is now experiencing pain because of talar subsidence. (*C*) Intraoperative view demonstrating a large fibrous build up of tissue limiting the range of motion of the ankle joint. (*D*) Technique of splitting the polyethylene piece is used to remove the polyethylene in the presence of talar subsidence. (*E*) The polyethylene piece on the back table after removal from the implant. (*F*) Intraoperative view after the removal of an Agility talar component and polyethylene piece. (*G, H*) Revision Agility low-profile talar component with the extended wings to cover the bony cortices of the talar body. (*I, J*) Intraoperative lateral and ankle mortise radiographs demonstrating a well-positioned revision Agility low-profile talar component with excellent talar cortex coverage.

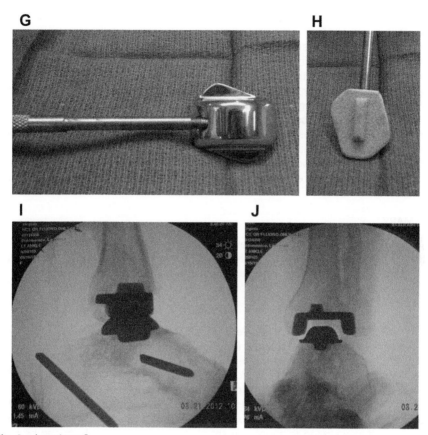

Fig. 8. (*continued*)

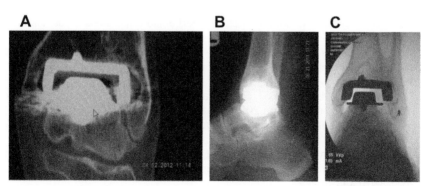

Fig. 9. (*A, B*) Preoperative CT scan and lateral radiograph demonstrating talar subsidence and bony overgrowth of the medial and lateral gutters. The bony overgrowth limited the range of motion of the ankle joint. (*C*) Intraoperative radiograph demonstrating a winged Agility talar low-profile component inserted and cemented with polymethyl methacrylate. The medial and lateral gutters were debrided decompressing the joint and allowing for increase in range of motion.

demonstrated bony clearing between the hydroxyapatite, implant, and bone in all the patients.

When performing a revisional-type surgery of TAR, replacement of the polyethylene meniscus may be necessary because of degradation of the component.[13] This is where implant design may affect the integrity of the device. Degradation may occur if the polyethylene does not fully conform to the bony components, if there is lack of capture by the other components to guide the polyethylene, or if it is larger than the surface of the tibial component.[34] Brooke and coworkers[17] in a case review of two patients undergoing revisional procedures for prior TAR noted deterioration specifically at the superiolateral aspect of the polyethylene piece in both patients, necessitating its removal. In addition to removal of the polyethylene, the same authors also recommended augmenting the revisional procedure by using a fibular-lengthening osteotomy if residual valgus deformity was present.

SUMMARY

Studies have demonstrated that the new generation of TAR systems provides superior patient satisfaction outcomes compared with prior systems and with ankle arthrodesis.[2] Ideally, a plantargrade foot type provides the optimal setting for application of TAR, and adjunctive procedures may be necessary to rectify concomitant biomechanical factors. If there is failure to address these areas, revisional procedures may be required.

A variety of TAR systems are available, and each has its own assets and pitfalls. When revisional or redo surgery is required, the standard main procedures consist of either joint arthrodesis or partial-total replacement of the implant. Additionally, soft tissue or bony debridement may prove useful for short-term or initial treatment. Arthrodesis is the modality chosen when there is inadequate bone stock or severe soft tissue compromise at the joint. A variety of methods to this procedure as previously described can be applied. Creativity can be used when exploring the implant replacement route, because it has been demonstrated that replacement of isolated or total implants can be performed with success, and hybridization of different implant systems.

REFERENCES

1. Raikin SM, Rampuri V. An approach to failed ankle arthrodesis. Foot Ankle Clin 2008;13:401–16.
2. Kwon DG, Chung CY, Park MS, et al. Arthroplasty versus arthrodesis for end-stage ankle arthritis: decision analysis using Markov model. Int Orthop 2011; 35:1647–53.
3. Spirit AA, Assal M, Hansen ST. Complications and failure after total ankle arthroplasty. J Bone Joint Surg Am 2004;86:1172–8.
4. Henricson A, Carlsson A, Rydholm U. What is a revision of total ankle replacement? Foot Ankle Surg 2011;17:99–102.
5. Berkowitz MJ, Clare MP, Walling AK, et al. Salvage of failed total ankle arthroplasty with fusion using structural allograft and internal fixation. Foot Ankle Int 2011;32(5):493–502.
6. Conti SF, Yong YS. Complications of total ankle replacement. Foot Ankle Clin 2002;7:791–807.
7. DiDomenico LA, Anania MC. Total ankle replacements: an overview. Clin Podiatr Med Surg 2010;28:727–44.
8. Bauer G, Eberhardt O, Rosenbaum D, et al. Total ankle replacement. Review and critical analysis of the current status. Foot Ankle Surg 1996;2:119–26.

9. Karantana A, Hobson S, Dhar S. The Scandinavian total ankle replacement: survivorship at 5 and 8 years comparable to other series. Clin Orthop Relat Res 2010; 468:951–7.
10. Makwana NK, Morrison P, Jones CB, et al. Salvage operations after failed total ankle replacement. Foot 1995;5:180–4.
11. Bonnin M, Gaudot F, Laurent JR, et al. The Salto total ankle arthroplasty. Clin Orthop Relat Res 2011;469:225–36.
12. Stamatis ED, Myerson MS. How to avoid specific complications of total ankle replacement. Foot Ankle Clin 2002;7:765–89.
13. Henricson A, Knutson K, Lindahl J, et al. The AES total ankle replacement: a mid-term analysis of 93 cases. Foot Ankle Surg 2010;16:61–4.
14. Schuberth JM, McCourt MJ, Christensen JC. Interval changes in postoperative range of motion of Salto-talaris total ankle replacement. J Foot Ankle Surg 2011;50:562–5.
15. Kakkar R, Siddique MS. Stresses in the ankle joint and total ankle replacement design. Foot Ankle Surg 2011;17:58–63.
16. Seth A. A Review of the STAR prosthetic system and the biomechanical considerations in total ankle replacements. Foot Ankle Surg 2011;17:64–7.
17. Brooke BT, Harris NJ, Morgan S. Fibula lengthening osteotomy to correct valgus malalignment following total ankle arthroplasty. Foot Ankle Surg 2009. http://dx.doi.org/10.1016/j.fas.2009.11.002.
18. Tan KJ, Myerson MS. Planning correction of the varus ankle deformity with ankle replacement. Foot Ankle Clin 2012;17(1):103–15.
19. Harris NJ, Brooke BT, Sturdee S. A wear debris cyst following STAR total ankle replacement: surgical management. Foot Ankle Surg 2009;15:43–5.
20. Myerson MS, Won HY. Primary and revision total ankle replacement using custom designed prosthesis. Foot Ankle Clin 2008;13:521–38.
21. Steck JK, Anderson JB. Total ankle arthroplasty: indications and avoiding complications. Clin Podiatr Med Surg 2009;26:303–24.
22. Henricson A, Agren PH. Secondary surgery after total ankle replacement: the influence of preoperative hindfoot alignment. Foot Ankle Surg 2007;13:41–4.
23. Wood PL, Deakin S. Total ankle replacement: the results in 200 ankles. J Bone Joint Surg Br 2003;85:334–41.
24. Zhao H, Yang Y, Yu G, et al. A systematic review of outcome and failure rate of uncemented Scandinavian total ankle replacement. Int Orthop 2011;35:1751–8.
25. Anderson T, Rydholm U, Besjakov J, et al. Tibiotalocalcaneal fusion using retrograde intramedullary nails as a salvage procedure for failed total ankle prosthesis in rheumatoid arthritis: a report on 16 cases. Foot Ankle Surg 2005;11:143–7.
26. Doets HC, Zurcher AW. Salvage arthrodesis for failed total ankle arthroplasty: clinical outcome and influence of method of fixation on union rate in 18 ankles followed for 3-12 years. Acta Orthop 2010;81(1):142–7.
27. Bullens P, Malefijt M, Louwerens JW. Conversion of failed ankle arthroplasty to an arthrodesis technique using an arthrodesis nail and a cage filled with morsellized bone graft. Foot Ankle Surg 2010;16:101–4.
28. Carlsson A. Unsuccessful use of a titanium mesh cage in ankle arthrodesis: a report on three cases operated on due to a failed ankle replacement. J Foot Ankle Surg 2008;47(4):337–42.
29. Kharwadkar N, Harris NJ. Revision of STAR total ankle replacement to hybrid AES-STAR total ankle replacement: a report of two cases. Foot Ankle Surg 2009;15:101–5.

30. Cerrato R, Myerson MS. Total ankle replacement: the agility LP prosthesis. Foot Ankle Clin 2008;13:485–94.
31. DeVries JG, Berlet GC, Lee TH, et al. Revision total ankle replacement: an early look at agility to inbone. Foot Ankle Spec 2011;4(4):235–44.
32. Schuberth JM, Christensen JC, Rialson JA. Metal-reinforced cement augmentation for complex talar subsidence in failed total ankle arthroplasty. J Foot Ankle Surg 2011;50:766–72.
33. Shi K, Hayashida K, Hashimoto J, et al. Hydroxyapatite augmentation for bone atrophy in total ankle replacement in rheumatoid arthritis. J Foot Ankle Surg 2006;45(5):308–15.
34. Hintermann B, Valderrabano V. Total ankle replacement. Foot Ankle Clin 2003;8: 375–405.

Current Concepts and Techniques in Foot and Ankle Surgery

Pinch Graft Harvesting Technique for Surgical Closure of the Diabetic Foot

Crystal L. Ramanujam, DPM, MSc, Thomas Zgonis, DPM, FACFAS*

KEYWORDS

• Diabetic foot • Wound • Surgery • Pinch grafts • Skin grafts • Neuropathy

KEY POINTS

- Skin-grafting techniques have evolved over time with regard to choices in donor sites, harvesting, and postoperative management.
- Pinch grafting has served as a viable method for treatment of venous and diabetic ulcerations of the leg.
- Pinch grafts harvested from the non–weight-bearing plantar forefoot region provide for immediate primary closure of the donor site.
- Medical optimization, adequate vascularity, and noninfected wounds are necessary before any surgical intervention.

INTRODUCTION

Skin grafting remains a mainstay of treatment for diabetic wounds that cannot be closed primarily or through standard local wound care. This procedure dates back to ancient times, first mentioned in Sanskrit manuscripts in 3000 BC, yet was first published for healing of ulcerations in 1869.[1] The decision to use a skin graft depends on wound condition, location, size, and esthetic considerations.[2] Specific techniques for skin grafting have evolved over time with regard to choices in donor sites, harvesting, and postoperative management of both the donor and recipient sites. Options for expedited, definitive closure can be limited based on the nature and location of the wound, as often seen in diabetic patients presenting with soft tissue loss following surgical debridement for complex foot infections.[3] Pinch grafting has served as a viable method for treatment of venous and diabetic ulcerations of the leg[1]; however, the surgical approach consisting of both donor and recipient sites located in the foot is

Division of Podiatric Medicine and Surgery, Department of Orthopaedic Surgery, University of Texas Health Science Center at San Antonio, San Antonio, TX, USA
* Corresponding author. 7703 Floyd Curl Drive MSC 7776, San Antonio, TX 78229.
E-mail address: zgonis@uthscsa.edu

Clin Podiatr Med Surg 29 (2012) 585–588
http://dx.doi.org/10.1016/j.cpm.2012.07.004
0891-8422/12/$ – see front matter © 2012 Elsevier Inc. All rights reserved.

unique. A case is presented illustrating the technique for pinch grafting harvested from the plantar forefoot to address a chronic diabetic foot ulceration.

CASE REPORT

A 34-year-old woman presented to the outpatient clinic with a right foot chronic ulceration to the plantar medial arch. The granular wound measured 4.0 × 1.5 × 0.3 cm without clinical or radiographic evidence of infection. The patient had undergone extensive surgical debridement for a foot abscess 2.5 months prior. She had been closely followed in a wound-care clinic for negative pressure wound therapy, serial wound debridement, and appropriate offloading. The patient had been maintained on oral amoxicillin-clavulanate based on intraoperative soft tissue cultures positive for group B *Streptococcus*. Her medical history included uncontrolled diabetes mellitus with peripheral neuropathy, hypertension, and hyperlipidemia. Noninvasive vascular testing showed no evidence of arterial occlusive disease to the affected foot. Because of the long duration of the wound despite consistent local wound care, definitive surgical wound closure was offered to the patient, including and not limited to skin grafting.

The patient was medically optimized by her primary care physician before surgery. Intravenous sedation with local anesthesia was administered to the patient in the operating room setting. Recipient wound bed preparation was performed to stimulate healthy bleeding via curettage and hydrosurgical debridement. The remaining 4 × 1-cm wound had no infection or necrosis and had a completely granular base. At the plantar aspect of the ipsilateral forefoot, just distal to the metatarsal heads, the donor site was marked with 2 semi-elliptical converging lines where the multiple pinch grafts were going to be harvested. The donor skin was infiltrated with 3 mL of 1% lidocaine with epinephrine and then using a 4-mm punch biopsy instrument, 11 separate pinch grafts were obtained through full-thickness skin, avoiding subcutaneous fat. The grafts were placed in saline temporarily while the remaining skin at the donor site was sharply excised in elliptical fashion following the previous markings. Primary closure of the donor site was performed using nonabsorbable suture in simple interrupted technique without tension. All 11 pinch grafts were carefully placed into the recipient wound bed at approximately 2-mm intervals, filling the defect. Topical thrombin was applied to the grafted site followed by a bolster-type dressing consisting of nonadherent gauze and saline-moistened sponges secured in place by skin staples and dry gauze dressing (**Fig. 1**).

The bolster dressing was removed 3 weeks later. After immobilization of the foot in a well-padded posterior splint for 3 additional weeks, the recipient and donor sites had completely healed. The patient was transitioned to weight bearing as tolerated in a surgical shoe, then gradually progressed into regular shoe gear without complications.

DISCUSSION

Classification of skin grafts includes 2 types: split-thickness skin that contains a variable thickness of dermis, whereas full-thickness skin contains the entire dermis. Full-thickness skin grafts are ideal for small, well-vascularized wounds.[4] They also retain more of the characteristics of normal skin, including texture, color, and thickness in addition to undergoing less contraction while healing. In contrast, split-thickness skin grafts can tolerate less-ideal conditions for survival, can be used in larger wounds, and have a wider range of application. Unfortunately, split- thickness skin grafts are more fragile and undergo significant contracture during healing.[2]

Pinch grafting as an alternative to full skin grafting was first described by J.S. Davis in 1914.[3] His original method involved lifting the skin with a needle and cutting the graft

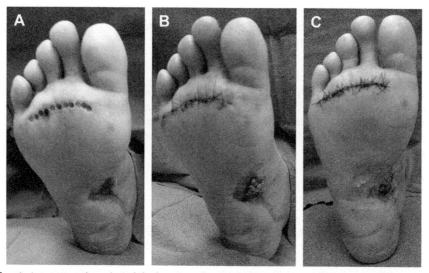

Fig. 1. Intraoperative view (*A*) showing the harvested pinch-grafting site distal to the plantar aspect of the metatarsal heads and application at the recipient area of the ipsilateral foot (*B*). Clinical view at the first postoperative visit showing healing without any complications (*C*).

longitudinally with a scalpel. This procedure has also been termed "punch grafting" when the graft is harvested using a punch biopsy instrument. Pinch grafting has been studied extensively for chronic leg ulcerations of many etiologies, including diabetic neuropathic wounds.[1,3] Because pinch grafting is a form of full-thickness skin grafting, a major advantage is that these grafts resist pressure better than their split-thickness counterparts, thus making them useful for wound coverage at the plantar aspect of the foot.

In this case report, primary wound closure was not an option because of the wound dimensions and location with lack of pliable surrounding skin. Split-thickness skin grafting was considered; however, an alternate method that could eliminate formation of an additional wound at the leg or thigh was more optimal. Full-thickness skin harvested from the plantar forefoot region provided for immediate primary closure of the donor site without any tension. Furthermore, the donor site, which was located at a non–weight-bearing location of the plantar forefoot, allowed for skin replacement that most resembled the original skin properties of the recipient location. This attribute enhances the function and durability of the wound closure.

Medical optimization and adequate vascularity should be established before skin grafting.[2] Attention to glycemic control and improved nutritional status are vital components to successful wound healing.[5,6] A wound environment that is free of infection in both the soft tissue and bone is required when considering skin grafting. Adequate debridement of the wound base is critical to reducing the bioburden and risk of future infection. A recipient bed that contains a bacterial concentration greater than 10^5 organisms per gram of tissue will not support a skin graft.[7] Dressings for pinch grafting traditionally incorporate paraffin and saline-moistened gauze followed with a hydrocellular foam layer and/or compressive dressing.[1,3] The bolster dressing used in this case presentation provides a nonadherent surface adjacent to the pinch grafting and also prevents motion at the graft-wound interface, thereby promoting graft take.[2] Posterior splint or casting techniques are helpful when treating the plantar surface of the foot and further eliminate motion. After healing at the donor and recipient sites, appropriate diabetic shoe gear should be considered for patients with diabetic neuropathy to prevent future ulceration.

SUMMARY

Pinch grafting is a relatively simple, reliable, and quick technique that can be used for treatment of certain foot wounds in the diabetic population. Harvesting of these grafts can be performed at the plantar forefoot in a non–weight-bearing location to minimize donor site morbidity and to provide similar tissue when addressing difficult-to-heal diabetic foot wounds.

REFERENCES

1. Oien RF, Håkansson A, Hansen BU, et al. Pinch grafting of chronic leg ulcers in primary care: fourteen years' experience. Acta Derm Venereol 2002;82(4):275–8.
2. Ramanujam CL, Stapleton JJ, Kilpadi KL, et al. Split-thickness skin grafts for closure of diabetic foot and ankle wounds: a retrospective review of 83 patients. Foot Ankle Spec 2010;3(5):231–40.
3. Oien RF, Hansen BU, Håkansson A. Pinch grafting of leg ulcers in primary care. Acta Derm Venereol 1998;78(6):438–9.
4. Mendez-Eastman S. Full-thickness skin grafting: a procedural review. Plast Surg Nurs 2004;24(2):41–5.
5. Thourani VH, Ingram WL, Feliciano DV. Factors affecting success of split thickness skin grafts in the modern burn unit. J Trauma 2003;54(3):562–8.
6. Mowlavi A, Andrews K, Milner S, et al. The effects of hyperglycemia on skin graft survival in the burn patient. Ann Plast Surg 2000;45(6):629–32.
7. Robson M, Krizek T. Predicting skin graft survival. J Trauma 1973;13(3):213–7.

An Overview of Bone Grafting Techniques for the Diabetic Charcot Foot and Ankle

Crystal L. Ramanujam, DPM, MSc[a], Zacharia Facaros, DPM[b],
Thomas Zgonis, DPM[a],*

KEYWORDS

- Bone graft • Autogenous bone • Allogenic bone • Diabetes mellitus • Charcot foot
- Reconstructive surgery

KEY POINTS

- Autogenous bone graft remains the gold standard because of complete histocompatibility but with certain limitations, including donor-site morbidity, limited supply, and increased surgical time.
- Allograft bone is typically categorized into osteoconductive and osteoinductive materials.
- Bone morphogenetic protein and other growth factors have been shown to be effective in bone healing.
- Combinations of autogenous and allograft bone graft have also shown success in complex diabetic Charcot foot and ankle reconstruction.

INTRODUCTION

Diabetic Charcot neuroarthropathy (CN) of the foot and ankle often presents a surgical challenge that requires careful consideration not only for the extent and type of deformity but also for the unique characteristics of the bone and soft tissue envelope involved with this patient population. Although the exact pathophysiologic mechanism of diabetic CN is unknown, current research has alluded to variations in bone physiology among patients with and without diabetes, peripheral neuropathy, and CN. These differences have contributed to changes in the way patients with diabetic CN are approached with regard to surgical reconstruction of the foot and ankle. Surgical techniques have evolved to include better fixation methods and designs, in addition to materials that can augment the construct for improved structural and functional outcomes. In this respect, bone grafting has gained an important role in the complex

[a] Division of Podiatric Medicine and Surgery, Department of Orthopaedic Surgery, University of Texas Health Science Center at San Antonio, 7703 Floyd Curl Drive, MSC 7776, San Antonio, TX 78229, USA; [b] Weil Foot & Ankle Institute, 1455 East Golf Road, Des Plaines, IL, USA
* Corresponding author.
E-mail address: zgonis@uthscsa.edu

Clin Podiatr Med Surg 29 (2012) 589–595
http://dx.doi.org/10.1016/j.cpm.2012.07.005
0891-8422/12/$ – see front matter © 2012 Elsevier Inc. All rights reserved.

reconstruction of diabetic CN foot and ankle deformities. Bone graft provides for the replacement of variable bone loss and enhancement of bone healing. Several choices exist among autograft, allograft, and bone graft substitutes, which can be tailored according to the overall clinical picture. An overview of several available options and specific applications is presented to maximize the surgeon's understanding of bone grafting in the diabetic CN foot and ankle.

AUTOGENOUS BONE GRAFTING FOR THE DIABETIC CHARCOT FOOT AND ANKLE

Autogenous bone graft remains the gold standard because of complete histocompatibility and no chance for disease transmission; however, its shortcomings include donor-site morbidity, limited supply, and increased surgical time.[1] Fred Albee[2] first described human autologous bone grafting in 1914 in which a patient's tibial bone was used for their spinal fusion. Today, types of autograft include cortical, cancellous, vascularized, and bone marrow aspirate. Autogenous cancellous graft is typically used as a nonstructural graft, frequently seen in arthrodesis. Cortical autograft provides structural support, therefore, allowing its use to span defects.

The most commonly used autogenous bone graft is the iliac crest (ICBG), which is harvested from either the anterior or posterior aspects and can be taken in the specific shape to span the defect.[3] For ankle arthrodesis in patients with CN, the ICBG is typically harvested from the contralateral side.[4] A study by El-Gafary and colleagues[5] on 20 patients with chronic CN deformities successfully used external fixation and corticocancellous bone graft harvested from the iliac crest for arthrodesis sites after debridement of necrotic and loose bone at the midfoot, hindfoot, and/or ankle. Shah and colleagues[6] used ICBG with monolateral external fixation or intramedullary nailing for ankle arthrodesis in 11 patients with chronic CN. Despite the advantages and versatility of ICBG, its complications at the donor site have been well reported, including infection, pain, sensory loss, hematoma formation, blood loss, and extended operating time.[3]

The disadvantages associated with ICBG have led to increased use of alternate harvest sites. Simon and colleagues[7] demonstrated successful tarsometatarsal arthrodesis using autologous cancellous graft harvested from the proximal tibia and internal fixation in 4 patients for the treatment of acute CN, whereas Deresh and Cohen[8] demonstrated successful midfoot and hindfoot arthrodesis using corticocancellous autograft harvested from the distal tibia for CN reconstruction.

The fibula can also be harvested for use as a cortical strut graft; however, postoperative complications in the literature have included differing degrees of pain and muscle weakness.[9] Jeong and colleagues[10] demonstrated stable CN ankle fusion using nonvascularized fibular graft with external fixation (**Fig. 1**). Free vascularized fibula graft provides better mechanical support because of earlier incorporation and has been reported in ankle arthrodesis for salvage following extensive osteomyelitis.[11] Small amounts of cancellous bone can be harvested from the calcaneus, with the lateral wall as the most common harvest site; however, other autogenous bone graft sites are considered better sources because of the limited amounts available for harvest and the possibility of interference with common arthrodesis sites in CN foot and ankle reconstruction.[12]

Surgery for CN often involves the removal of severely dislocated and fractured bone to produce a shortened yet stable foot for ambulation. This resected bone can be prepared intraoperatively via morselization and decortication for use as autograft at the index arthrodesis site. This technique precludes the need for a remote site of bone harvest and can be combined with allogenic bone graft to facilitate incorporation.

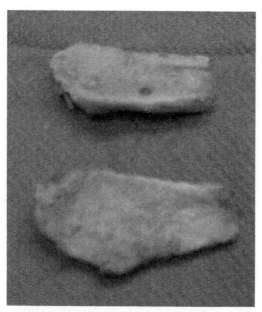

Fig. 1. Intraoperative clinical picture demonstrating the harvested autogenous distal fibula bone graft for incorporation at the diabetic Charcot ankle arthrodesis site. Please note the final outcome of the autogenous fibular graft, which has been resected in half for alignment and incorporation within the ankle joint.

Use of bone marrow aspirate (BMA) to stimulate skeletal repair originated with Goujon in 1869 where he observed the ability of autologous marrow to induce bone at heterotopic sites.[3] Bone marrow is most often aspirated from the iliac crest and then can be injected percutaneously to stimulate osteogenesis. A disadvantage of BMA includes only a limited supply of stem cells available in obtained samples; however, its high osteogenic potential makes it useful in combination with allograft materials such as those with an osteoconductive matrix. Pinzur[13] showed a combination of BMA with platelet rich plasma can be effective in foot arthrodesis for diabetic CN.

ALLOGENIC BONE GRAFTING FOR THE DIABETIC CHARCOT FOOT AND ANKLE

Sir William MacEwen introduced allografting in 1879 by replacing the proximal humerus in a young child with bone transplanted from other patients.[3] Allograft types include cancellous or cortical bone, cadaveric bone (typically fresh-frozen or freeze-dried), and demineralized and synthetic bone grafts. Joint preparation in diabetic CN foot ankle reconstruction typically leaves areas of extensive bone loss, particularly so in cases of superimposed osteomyelitis. Allograft has become a popular option for these large bone voids because of the often limited supply of autograft (**Fig. 2**). The use of structural allografts avoids the morbidity and extended surgical times associated with autogenous bone grafting.[14] These attributes are of increased importance among patients with diabetic CN who may already have comorbidities that can potentially compound surgical risk. Various techniques, including freeze-drying, liquid nitrogen freezing, and demineralizing, are used in processing allograft to decrease the risk of disease transmission and for storage purposes.[15] Cadaveric femoral head and iliac crest allografts are effective in major CN foot and ankle arthrodesis

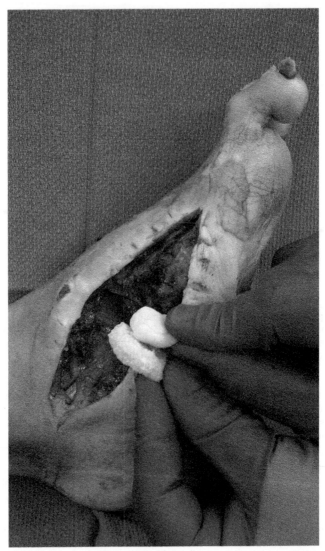

Fig. 2. Intraoperative clinical picture demonstrating an example of a combined osteoconductive and osteoinductive allogenic bone grafts for a diabetic Charcot midfoot reconstruction after a wide correctional midfoot osteotomy.

because of their availability and reliable structural support. Careful consideration should be made in the use of these allografts because the risk of an immune response can be heightened in patients with diabetes who are already immunocompromised.

Inorganic bioceramics, calcium phosphate and calcium sulfate, and hydroxyapatites are examples of bone graft substitutes. These products are readily available in unlimited quantities and useful for large bone defects and at autogenous bone graft donor sites. Their application in reconstruction of the diabetic CN foot and ankle has been limited to filling of bone voids and to augment other materials for onlay grafting. The use of a ceramic bone graft substitute comprised of calcium sulfate and hydroxyapatite has been reported for the direct delivery of antibiotics in the treatment of foot osteomyelitis; therefore, this technique may facilitate staged reconstruction for diabetic CN superimposed with osteomyelitis.[16]

Since the first description of bone morphogenetic proteins (BMPs) by Marshall Urist in the 1960s, several of these growth factors have proven effective in diabetic foot and ankle surgery.[17] In diabetic CN, demineralized bone matrix (DBM) is perhaps the most commonly used form of BMPs (**Fig. 3**). DBM products vary in the amounts and types of BMPs they contain, yet they can be easily combined with autologous or allogenic bone graft material for use in CN corrective arthrodesis and/or the treatment of nonunions.[18,19] Schuberth and colleagues[17] used BMPs in CN foot and ankle surgery for 10 patients whereby only 1 of these did not consolidate, which the investigators attributed to previous infection.

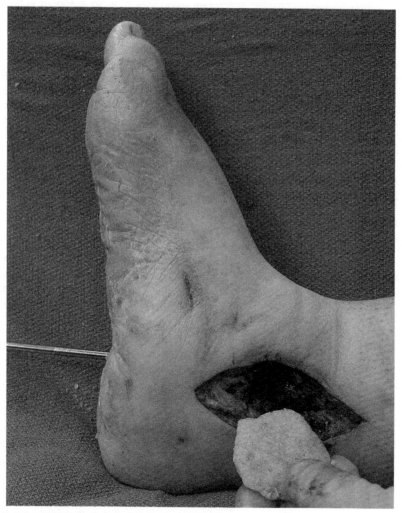

Fig. 3. Intraoperative clinical picture demonstrating an example of a DBM allogenic bone graft for incorporation at the diabetic Charcot ankle arthrodesis site.

The potential activity of certain allograft products is based on their combination with living osteogenic cells. Platelet gel concentrate or plasma is an autologous concentration of platelets involving multiple growth factors that can serve as a helpful adjunct in bone healing.[12] Intraoperatively, these platelet aggregates are obtained from the patient and produce platelet-rich plasma that can be combined with other bone graft material for fusion sites and platelet-poor plasma that can be applied on any existing wounds associated with the CN deformity to optimize healing.

Mesenchymal stem cells (MSCs) are multipotent connective tissue cells that can activate cell repair and provide the basis for an emerging market in bone substitution and repair. Mesenchymal cell-based bone allograft from cadaveric donors is comprised of morselized cancellous bone that is processed to reduce immunogenicity and maintains viable bone-forming cells. A recent study by Hollawell[20] presented successful fusion rates in hindfoot and ankle procedures using allograft cellular bone matrix as an alternative to autograft in 3 patients with diabetic CN. Lee and Mulder[21] also showed promising outcomes using MSCs as an autograft substitute in diabetic CN foot and ankle reconstruction for 7 patients; however, future larger clinical and randomized studies are needed to provide more conclusive results for this method.

Combinations of the aforementioned autogenous and allograft materials have also shown success in complex diabetic CN foot and ankle surgery. In diabetic CN midfoot arthrodesis, Deresh and Cohen[8] used cadaveric freeze-dried corticocancellous allograft bone and autograft harvested from the ipsilateral tibia for CN midfoot deformity. All cases demonstrated satisfactory arthrodesis within a period of 4 to 6 months. Myerson and colleagues[22] reported tibiocalcaneal fusion in 30 patients for the management of severe hindfoot and ankle deformities, including 26 patients with diabetic neuroarthropathy. The special properties associated with each type of graft in relation to bone structure and physiology provide surgeons creative approaches to establishing a stable, functional construct.

SUMMARY

As research grows to provide more answers to the underlying pathophysiology of diabetic CN of the foot and ankle, surgical technologies continue to evolve for better management of these complex cases. Unquestionably, autogenous and allogenic bone grafting plays an important role in reconstructive foot and ankle surgery. A clear understanding of the use of these versatile materials in the correct clinical setting may lead to more optimal outcomes in high-risk patients with diabetic CN.

REFERENCES

1. Khan SN, Cammisa FP Jr, Sandhu HS, et al. The biology of bone grafting. J Am Acad Orthop Surg 2005;13(1):77–86.
2. Albee FH. Transplantation of a portion of the tibia into the spine for Pott's disease. JAMA 1914;57:885.
3. Fitzgibbons TC, Hawks MA, McMullen ST, et al. Bone grafting in surgery about the foot and ankle: indications and techniques. J Am Acad Orthop Surg 2011; 19(2):112–20.
4. Zgonis T, Stapleton JJ, Jeffries LC, et al. Surgical treatment of Charcot neuropathy. AORN J 2008;87(5):971–86.
5. El-Gafary KA, Mostafa KM, Al-Adly WY. The management of Charcot joint disease affecting the ankle and foot by arthrodesis controlled by an Ilizarov frame: early results. J Bone Joint Surg Br 2009;91(10):1322–5.

6. Shah NS, De SD. Comparative analysis of uniplanar external fixator and retrograde intramedullary nailing for ankle arthrodesis in diabetic Charcot's neuroarthropathy. Indian J Orthop 2011;45(4):359–64.

7. Simon SR, Tejwani SG, Wilson DL, et al. Arthrodesis as an early alternative to nonoperative management of Charcot arthropathy of the diabetic foot. J Bone Joint Surg Am 2000;82-A(7):939–50.

8. Deresh GM, Cohen M. Reconstruction of the diabetic Charcot foot incorporating bone grafts. J Foot Ankle Surg 1996;35(5):474–88.

9. Gore DR, Gardner GM, Sepic SB, et al. Function following partial fibulectomy. Clin Orthop Relat Res 1987;220:206–10.

10. Jeong ST, Park HB, Hwang SC, et al. Use of intramedullary nonvascularized fibular graft with external fixation for revisional Charcot ankle fusion: a case report. J Foot Ankle Surg 2012;51(2):249–53.

11. Bishop AT, Wood MB, Sheetz KK. Arthrodesis of the ankle with a free vascularized autogenous bone graft. Reconstruction of segmental loss of bone secondary to osteomyelitis, tumor, or trauma. J Bone Joint Surg Am 1995;77(12):1867–75.

12. Anderson JJ. "Bone grafting and orthobiologics for reconstruction of the diabetic lower extremity". In: Zgonis T, editor. Surgical reconstruction of the diabetic foot and ankle. Philadelphia: Lippincott Williams & Wilkins; 2009. p. 283–99.

13. Pinzur MS. Use of platelet-rich concentrate and bone marrow aspirate in high-risk patients with Charcot arthropathy of the foot. Foot Ankle Int 2009;30(2):124–7.

14. Neufeld SK, Uribe J, Myerson MS. Use of structural allograft to compensate for bone loss in arthrodesis of the foot and ankle. Foot Ankle Clin 2002;7(1):1–17.

15. Boyce T, Edwards J, Scarborough N. Allograft bone. The influence of processing on safety and performance. Orthop Clin North Am 1999;30:571–81.

16. Karr JC. Management in the wound-care center outpatient setting of a diabetic patient with forefoot osteomyelitis using Cerament Bone Void Filler impregnated with vancomycin: off-label use. J Am Podiatr Med Assoc 2011;101(3):259–64.

17. Schuberth JM, DiDomenico LA, Mendicino RW. The utility and effectiveness of bone morphogenetic protein in foot and ankle surgery. J Foot Ankle Surg 2009; 48(3):309–14.

18. Pacaccio DJ, Stern SF. Demineralized bone matrix: basic science and clinical applications. Clin Podiatr Med Surg 2005;22(4):599–606.

19. Bevilacqua NJ, Stapleton JJ. Advanced foot and ankle fixation techniques in patients with diabetes. Clin Podiatr Med Surg 2011;28(4):661–71.

20. Hollawell SM. Allograft cellular bone matrix as an alternative to autograft in hindfoot and ankle fusion procedures. J Foot Ankle Surg 2012;51:222–5.

21. Lee DK, Mulder GD. Stem cell applications in diabetic Charcot foot and ankle reconstructive surgery. Wounds 2010;22(9):226–9.

22. Myerson MS, Alvarez RG, Lam PW. Tibiocalcaneal arthrodesis for the management of severe ankle and hindfoot deformities. Foot Ankle Int 2000;21:643–50.

Index

Note: Page numbers of article titles are in **boldface** type.

Clin Podiatr Med Surg 29 (2012) 597–603
http://dx.doi.org/10.1016/S0891-8422(12)00121-8
0891-8422/12/$ – see front matter © 2012 Elsevier Inc. All rights reserved.

podiatric.theclinics.com

United States Postal Service

Statement of Ownership, Management, and Circulation
(All Periodicals Publications Except Requestor Publications)

1. Publication Title	2. Publication Number	3. Filing Date
Clinics in Podiatric Medicine & Surgery	0 0 0 - 7 0 7	9/14/12

4. Issue Frequency	5. Number of Issues Published Annually	6. Annual Subscription Price
Jan, Apr, Jul, Oct	4	$292.00

7. Complete Mailing Address of Known Office of Publication (Not printer) (Street, city, county, state, and ZIP+4®)

Elsevier Inc.
360 Park Avenue South
New York, NY 10010-1710

Contact Person
Stephen R. Bushing
Telephone (Include area code)
215-239-3688

8. Complete Mailing Address of Headquarters or General Business Office of Publisher (Not printer)

Elsevier Inc., 360 Park Avenue South, New York, NY 10010-1710

9. Full Names and Complete Mailing Addresses of Publisher, Editor, and Managing Editor (Do not leave blank)

Publisher (Name and complete mailing address)

Kim Murphy, Elsevier, Inc., 1600 John F. Kennedy Blvd. Suite 1800, Philadelphia, PA 19103-2899

Editor (Name and complete mailing address)

Patrick Manley, Elsevier, Inc., 1600 John F. Kennedy Blvd. Suite 1800, Philadelphia, PA 19103-2899

Managing Editor (Name and complete mailing address)

Barbara Cohen - Kligerman, Elsevier, Inc., 1600 John F. Kennedy Blvd. Suite 1800, Philadelphia, PA 19103-2899

10. Owner (Do not leave blank. If the publication is owned by a corporation, give the name and address of the corporation immediately followed by the names and addresses of all stockholders owning or holding 1 percent or more of the total amount of stock. If not owned by a corporation, give the names and addresses of the individual owners. If owned by a partnership or other unincorporated firm, give its name and address as well as those of each individual owner. If the publication is published by a nonprofit organization, give its name and address.)

Full Name	Complete Mailing Address
Wholly owned subsidiary of	1600 John F. Kennedy Blvd., Ste. 1800
Reed/Elsevier, US holdings	Philadelphia, PA 19103-2899

11. Known Bondholders, Mortgagees, and Other Security Holders Owning or Holding 1 Percent or More of Total Amount of Bonds, Mortgages, or Other Securities. If none, check box ☐ None

Full Name	Complete Mailing Address
N/A	

12. Tax Status (For completion by nonprofit organizations authorized to mail at nonprofit rates) (Check one)
The purpose, function, and nonprofit status of this organization and the exempt status for federal income tax purposes:
☐ Has Not Changed During Preceding 12 Months
☐ Has Changed During Preceding 12 Months (Publisher must submit explanation of change with this statement)

PS Form 3526, September 2007 (Page 1 of 3 (Instructions Page 3)) PSN 7530-01-000-9931 **PRIVACY NOTICE:** See our Privacy policy in www.usps.com

---

13. Publication Title		14. Issue Date for Circulation Data Below
Clinics in Podiatric Medicine & Surgery		July 2012

15. Extent and Nature of Circulation		Average No. Copies Each Issue During Preceding 12 Months	No. Copies of Single Issue Published Nearest to Filing Date
a. Total Number of Copies (Net press run)		804	632
b. Paid Circulation (By Mail and Outside the Mail)	(1) Mailed Outside-County Paid Subscriptions Stated on PS Form 3541. (Include paid distribution above nominal rate, advertiser's proof copies, and exchange copies)	513	470
	(2) Mailed In-County Paid Subscriptions Stated on PS Form 3541 (Include paid distribution above nominal rate, advertiser's proof copies, and exchange copies)		
	(3) Paid Distribution Outside the Mails Including Sales Through Dealers and Carriers, Street Vendors, Counter Sales, and Other Paid Distribution Outside USPS®	43	49
	(4) Paid Distribution by Other Classes Mailed Through the USPS (e.g. First-Class Mail®)		
c. Total Paid Distribution (Sum of 15b (1), (2), (3), and (4))	►	556	519
d. Free or Nominal Rate Distribution (By Mail and Outside the Mail)	(1) Free or Nominal Rate Outside-County Copies Included on PS Form 3541	79	74
	(2) Free or Nominal Rate In-County Copies Included on PS Form 3541		
	(3) Free or Nominal Rate Copies Mailed at Other Classes Through the USPS (e.g. First-Class Mail)		
	(4) Free or Nominal Rate Distribution Outside the Mail (Carriers or other means)		
e. Total Free or Nominal Rate Distribution (Sum of 15d (1), (2), (3) and (4))	►	79	74
f. Total Distribution (Sum of 15c and 15e)	►	635	593
g. Copies not Distributed (See instructions to publishers #4 (page #3))	►	169	39
h. Total (Sum of 15f and g)	►	804	632
i. Percent Paid (15c divided by 15f times 100)		87.56%	87.52%

16. Publication of Statement of Ownership

☑ If the publication is a general publication, publication of this statement is required. Will be printed ☐ Publication not required
in the October 2012 issue of this publication.

17. Signature and Title of Editor, Publisher, Business Manager, or Owner	Date
[signature] Stephen R. Bushing – Inventory/Distribution Coordinator	September 14, 2012

I certify that all information furnished on this form is true and complete. I understand that anyone who furnishes false or misleading information on this form or who omits material or information requested on the form may be subject to criminal sanctions (including fines and imprisonment) and/or civil sanctions (including civil penalties).

PS Form 3526, September 2007 (Page 2 of 3)

Moving?

Make sure your subscription moves with you!

To notify us of your new address, find your **Clinics Account Number** (located on your mailing label above your name), and contact customer service at:

Email: journalscustomerservice-usa@elsevier.com

800-654-2452 (subscribers in the U.S. & Canada)
314-447-8871 (subscribers outside of the U.S. & Canada)

Fax number: 314-447-8029

Elsevier Health Sciences Division
Subscription Customer Service
3251 Riverport Lane
Maryland Heights, MO 63043

*To ensure uninterrupted delivery of your subscription, please notify us at least 4 weeks in advance of move.

Printed and bound by CPI Group (UK) Ltd, Croydon, CR0 4YY

03/10/2024

01040456-0011